Amazing

Inch Loss Plan

Rosemary Conley CBE is the UK's most successful diet and fitness expert. Her diet and fitness books, videos and DVDs have consistently topped the bestseller lists with combined sales approaching nine million copies.

Rosemary has also presented more than 400 cookery programmes on television and has hosted several of her own TV series on BBC and ITV including Slim to Win with Rosemary Conley, which was first broadcast in ITV Central and Thames Valley regions in 2007, with a new series in 2008.

In 1999 Rosemary was made a Deputy Lieutenant of Leicestershire. In 2001 she was given the Freedom of the City of Leicester, and in 2004 she was awarded a CBE in the Queen's New Year Honours List for 'services to the fitness and diet industries'.

Together with her husband, Mike Rimmington, Rosemary runs five companies: Rosemary Conley Diet and Fitness Clubs, which operates an award-winning national network of almost 200 franchises running around 2000 classes weekly; Quorn House Publishing Ltd, which publishes Rosemary Conley Diet and Fitness magazine; Quorn House Media Ltd, which runs rosemaryconley.tv, an online TV channel; Rosemary Conley Licences Ltd; and Rosemary Conley Enterprises.

Rosemary has a daughter, Dawn, from her first marriage. Rosemary, Mike and Dawn are all committed Christians.

Also by Rosemary Conley

Rosemary Conley's Hip and Thigh Diet
Rosemary Conley's Complete Hip and Thigh Diet
Rosemary Conley's Inch Loss Plan
Rosemary Conley's Hip and Thigh Diet Cookbook
(with Patricia Bourne)
Rosemary Conley's Metabolism Booster Diet
Rosemary Conley's Whole Body Programme
Rosemary Conley's New Hip and Thigh Diet Cookbook
(with Patricia Bourne)
Shape Up for Summer
Rosemary Conley's Beach Body Plan
Rosemary Conley's Flat Stomach Plan
Be Slim! Be Fit!
Rosemary Conley's Complete Flat Stomach Plan
Rosemary Conley's New Body Plan
Rosemary Conley's New Inch Loss Plan
Rosemary Conley's Low Fat Cookbook
Rosemary Conley's Red Wine Diet
Rosemary Conley's Low Fat Cookbook Two
Rosemary Conley's Eat Yourself Slim
Rosemary Conley's Step by Step Low Fat Cookbook
Rosemary Conley's Gi Jeans Diet
Rosemary Conley's Ultimate Gi Jeans Diet
Rosemary Conley's Gi Hip and Thigh Diet
Slim to Win Diet and Cookbook

Rosemary Conley's
Amazing
Inch Loss Plan

Lose a stone in a month!

Northumberland County Council	
3 0132 02095370 4	
Askews & Holts	Feb-2012
613.25	£6.99

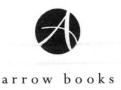

arrow books

First published in the United Kingdom by Century in 2010
This revised edition published by Arrow in 2011

10 9 8 7 6 5 4 3 2 1

Copyright © Rosemary Conley Enterprises 2010, 2011

Rosemary Conley has asserted her right under the Copyright, Designs and
Patents Act, 1988 to be identified as the author of this work

This book is sold subject to the condition that it shall not, by way of trade or
otherwise, be lent, resold, hired out, or otherwise circulated without the
publisher's prior consent in any form of binding or cover other than that in which
it is published and without a similar condition including this condition being
imposed on the subsequent purchaser

Arrow
Random House UK Limited
20 Vauxhall Bridge Road, London SW1V 2SA

Addresses for companies within The Random House Group Ltd can be found at
www.randomhouse.co.uk/offices.htm

The Random House UK Limited Reg. No. 954009

A CIP catalogue record for this book is available from the British Library

ISBN 9780099543145

Front cover photograph by Alan Olley
Exercise photography by Alan Olley
Edited by Jan Bowmer
Designed by Roger Walker

The Random House Group Limited supports The Forest Stewardship Council
(FSC), the leading international forest certification organisation. All our titles
that are printed on Greenpeace approved FSC certified paper carry the FSC logo.
Our paper procurement policy can be found at www.rbooks.co.uk/environment

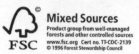

Mixed Sources
Product group from well-managed
forests and other controlled sources
www.fsc.org Cert no. TT-COC-2139
© 1996 Forest Stewardship Council

Printed and bound in Great Britain by
CPI Bookmarque, Croydon, Surrey CR0 4TD

The diet in this book is based on sound healthy eating
principles. However, it is important to check with your
doctor or medical practitioner before following any
weight-reducing plan.

Contents

Acknowledgements

This new edition of my *Amazing Inch Loss Plan* would not have been possible without the help of my great team.

In my original *Amazing Inch Loss Plan* book I thanked the many people who had helped me with different aspects of the book: chef Dean Simpole-Clarke for the recipes; Sue White and Bridget Key for running the diet trial; Mary Morris for her expertise and guidance on the exercises and, in this revised book, her tremendous technical knowledge and input in the 'Are you doing your five-a-week?' chapter; Caroline Whiting, Head of Training at Rosemary Conley Diet and Fitness Clubs, for her help on how to get folk motivated; and Dr Susan Jebb, an eminent nutrition scientist, for her expertise and guidance on the nutritional principles that I follow.

A big thank you to our wonderfully talented franchisees who run Rosemary Conley Diet and Fitness Clubs and who have supported their members as they followed the Amazing Inch Loss Plan in our classes over the last year. Without them I would not have had the thrill and privilege of meeting, a week before this book went to print, four spectacularly successful slimmers who had lost 37 stone between them in the last ten months on my Amazing Inch Loss Plan! Eve Leonard, Stephanie Hughes, Carl Williams and Michael Hutchinson have proved beyond doubt that this diet and fitness plan works and are now among my Slimmers of the Year for 2011.

This latest version of my *Amazing Inch Loss Plan* has been greatly extended by the inclusion of an extra diet plan: my Amazing Inch Loss Plan Solo Slim diet. Based on the highly nutritious and very convenient ready meals which we have created, I have produced a diet plan that has been tried and tested, both by some new dieters and others who had been dieting for a while but who had seen their weight-loss progress stalling. This diet is included in this book for the first time and I hope it will give hope to any struggling dieter! I would like to thank Teresa Lewis, our Solo Slim Foods Manager, for her help in selecting new flavours and products for the range in order to maximise the choice for you, the reader. I must again thank Sue White, our researcher, who undertook and supervised this latest trial, and to all the trialists who participated. A big thank you, also, to my PA, Louise Jones, for deciphering my endless ramblings when I was dictating and writing the many additions to this book; to Anja Zeman for calculating the calories of all the menus; and to Sian Cartwright for her contribution to the 'Eating out on a diet' chapter.

Thanks also to Gemma Binch and the production team at www.rosemaryconley.tv for recording the 28 days of workouts that are included on the website for you, the reader, to follow, day by day. This entailed a lot of work and this innovative advance in technology has enabled this book to come to life. The production team also recorded interviews with some of our trial dieters so that you can see their progress on this diet.

Most of all, I want to thank my editor, Jan Bowmer, with whom I have had the privilege of working for over 20 years. The reformatting of this book from its original presentation was a mammoth task and Jan is a master for detail and has the most logical brain, which makes my job so much easier. Jan, you are a total star! Thank you also to Roger Walker for designing the book in just the way I hoped it would be.

Finally, thank you to all my readers. I hope that you will find this book does exactly what you want it to and that you will see a slimmer, fitter you emerging after just 28 days, and beyond. And I hope you will go on to enjoy further benefits as you continue to follow the principles of this book.

Useful information

Body weight conversions

Pound (lb)	Stone (st)	Kilogram (kg)
1		0.5
2		1
3		1.4
4		1.8
5		2.3
6		2.7
7	½	3.2
8		3.6
9		4.1
10		4.5
11		5
12		5.4
13		5.9
14	1	6.3
28	2	12.7

Spoon measures

1 teaspoon = 5ml	
1 dessertspoon = 10ml	
1 tablespoon = 15ml	

Abbreviations and symbols used

lb	pound
g	gram
kg	kilogram
st	stone
ml	millilitre
in	inch
ft	foot
mm	millimetre
cm	centimetre
kcal	calorie
tsp	teaspoon
tbsp	tablespoon
dsp	dessertspoon
✔	suitable for vegetarians
❄	suitable for home freezing
P	high protein food option

Visit www.rosemaryconley.com
for more diet and fitness advice.

1 How to lose weight fast

If you want to lose weight faster than ever before, then this is the diet for you! Just look at the successful slimmers featured on the back cover of this book and in the photographs inside to see how amazingly this diet and fitness plan works. Stephanie Hughes lost 12 stone in 10 months. Michael Hutchinson lost 10 stone in 10 months. Carl Williams lost 9 stone in six months and 22 year-old student Eve Leonard lost 5st 10lb in nine months.

So, would *you* like to start by losing a stone in a month? Well, providing you have a reasonable amount of weight to lose, you should be able to do just that. Fifty volunteers who followed the diet over a four-week period lost 50 stone between them and that's why I can make such a bold claim that you can indeed **lose a stone in a month**.

Our 50-strong trial team consisted of men and women of various ages and weights. The youngest participant was eighteen-year-old Jane Gillespie, who weighed in at 11st 5lb at the start of the trial. At the end of the four weeks Jane weighed 9st 12lb, having dropped two dress sizes in one month. The oldest participant was Jenny Winning, who was 70 years old at the time of the trial. Jenny lost 13¾lb in four weeks.

This diet *works* and, providing you stick to it to the letter, you will see incredible results on the scales. And if you do the recommended daily exercises and aerobic challenges, not only will you lose weight but you will also shed an amazing number of inches from around your body.

My original *Amazing Inch Loss Plan* book was published in January 2010 and went straight into the bestseller charts. This new edition, which is published in a smaller format so it's handy to put in your handbag or briefcase, includes testimonials from many successful slimmers who have followed the diet in the original book or at a Rosemary Conley Diet and Fitness Club.

The Amazing Inch Loss Plan diet was introduced into Rosemary Conley Diet and Fitness Clubs in January 2010 and in the 17 years that the clubs have been in operation our franchisees say they have never witnessed such astonishing weight losses among their class members. I've seen this too at my own classes, which I still teach on Monday evenings, and I can't explain the excitement I feel when I see my members physically shrinking in front of my very eyes, week after week.

So what makes this diet different?

The Amazing Inch Loss Plan is a fairly strict, calorie-controlled, healthy eating plan combined with a structured aerobic and toning programme. The eating plan is based on 1200 calories a day for the first two weeks. This results in a fantastic weight loss after just 14 days, giving participants a massive boost and the motivation to continue for the next two weeks on a more generous 1400 calories per day. From week five, the recommended calorie allowance is based on an individual's age, gender and weight, which will enable them to carry on losing weight at a steady pace of 1–3lb a week depending on how strictly they stick to their calorie allowance and how determined they are to exercise on a daily basis. It's a classic case of the harder you try, the greater the results.

Work out with me

One exciting new development with this updated version of the Amazing Inch Loss Plan is that we have taken the daily exercises from the original book and filmed them for our internet television channel (www.rosemaryconley.tv). So, while you are following the 28-day plan you can tune in and work out with me each day as I demonstrate the toning exercises that will reshape your body. The exercises are progressive so that everyone can do them, and the programme is designed in such a way to enable you to advance at a very comfortable level and achieve maximum strength and mobility by the end of the 28-day period. To enjoy this unique service, all you have to do is log on to www.rosemaryconley.tv/ailpDay1, ailpDay2, etc., and of course it's absolutely free. Try to follow the exercises in sequence as they have been carefully planned to work all the main muscles in the body in the safest and most effective way.

To maximise your weight loss you will also need to undertake some aerobic exercise on a regular basis. Aerobic exercise is quite different from the toning exercises that accompany this book as it works the heart and lungs and burns body fat. On each day of this plan you will see that I suggest an aerobic challenge, which could be going for a brisk walk or a swim, working out at a fitness class – such as a Rosemary Conley Diet and Fitness Club class – or to an aerobic fitness DVD. All my fitness DVDs are suitable for this purpose, although my Real Results Workout is particularly effective. The benefit of using the aerobic workout from one of my DVDs is that it targets the whole body so it will not only increase your fitness, but give you a great shape too. See www.rosemaryconley.com to check the

'My weight would not budge until I followed this diet. I don't feel I've been on a diet but a healthy eating plan that I plan to keep following. I feel so much better and can now wear clothes I had "grown out of"! Thank you!'
Gillian Betts

selection of DVDs available. If you have any physical restrictions, you can try my Ultimate Whole Body Workout, which includes an aerobic chair exercise programme.

High-protein eating

More and more people are choosing to cut down on carbohydrates, and my Amazing Inch Loss Plan was the first of my diets to include some high-protein, low-carbohydrate options. In the diet trial, it was interesting to note that the people who followed the high-protein options lost just as much weight as those who chose the high-carbohydrate alternatives, so it comes down to personal choice. Both options contain lots of filling foods. The high-carbohydrate menus are based on low-Gi foods, which release energy slowly and keep you feeling fuller for longer, while high-protein meals have been proven to have a high satiety value. The result is that my dieters have found it surprisingly easy to survive on as few as 1200 calories a day without feeling hungry.

This diet is medically approved and offers a vast array of different foods for you to eat.

Solo Slim

My Solo Slim® range of ready meals was launched in 2010. All the meals are low in fat, calorie controlled, contain no E numbers and are totally healthy. The meals are prepared in such a way that you do not even need to refrigerate them and they have a shelf life of up to 12 months. They are the perfect answer for those occasions when you don't know what to eat in the evening or want something quick when you get home from work. Alternatively, you can base your diet around them, eating a different flavoured soup or ready meal at lunchtime and a different ready meal each evening. These products are only available as part of a Rosemary Conley healthy food box. Alternatively, you may be able to purchase them via our classes. You can choose which meals you want to include in your box and order them online from www.rosemaryconley.com or by phone to ensure you get exactly what you want delivered directly to your home.

'Both me and my doctor are very happy! Losing so much weight in just a month, and so easily, is amazing!'
Bill Wiltshire

In this book I have included a Solo Slim diet based on these ready meals. This takes all the choice and decision-making of what to eat out of your daily routine, as all you have to do is open the packet, heat it in the microwave or empty the contents into a saucepan and cook up some vegetables of your choice and, hey presto, you have your calorie-controlled, ready prepared meal. For many people, this makes dieting easier and more effective as there is no room for error when calculating food quantities and portion sizes.

To prove the effectiveness of the Amazing Inch Loss Plan Solo Slim diet, we carried out another trial where dieters were asked to live on Solo Slim® foods for one month, just adding fruit, additional vegetables or salad and their chosen breakfast menu from the options given. The results were astonishing. The trial dieters found the diet easy to follow, incredibly convenient and they loved the fact that they didn't have to spend time preparing the meals. Even those participants with not a great deal of weight to lose were amazed at how fast the pounds dropped away. It was just so easy.

It's up to you whether you want to follow the Solo Slim diet in its entirety or you just want to incorporate the occasional Solo Slim meal into your free choice diet. After you have reached your ideal weight, Solo Slim can prove extremely helpful in maintaining your new figure. Using Solo Slim meals for, say, just two days a week could be enough to allow you to eat reasonably normally for the rest of the time providing you stick with your new low-fat way of eating and active way of life. All of the Solo Slim menus are personally selected and tasted by me and they really do give you a very substantial and delicious meal, either at lunchtime or in the evening. And as each meal is calorie controlled and low fat, you know exactly what you can accompany it with to keep within your calorie allowance and ensure maximum slimming success.

My daily motivational tips will keep your willpower topped up and, along the journey, you will learn how to speed up your weight loss, tone up your muscles and turn your body into a 'fat burner' rather than a 'fat storer' so you can stay slim without ever having to diet again.

You really have nothing to lose but your weight so what are you waiting for?

2 The diet trial

Over the years I have held several trials to test my diets. It's helpful for me to have ordinary folk who lead regular lives try out my eating plans, because it provides real proof that the diet in question works and is easy to follow. Their comments, observations and experiences then enable me to tweak the diet if necessary to make it more practical and therefore more effective in the long term.

I had already carried out two previous trials to determine how much weight it was possible to lose safely in two weeks on an eating plan based on 1200 calories a day. With this Amazing Inch Loss Plan, I wanted to see if men and women alike could continue for a second two-week period on a relatively low number of calories, in the hope of proving that it was possible to lose a stone in four weeks. Prior to creating this strict four-week diet, I took professional advice from Dr Susan Jebb, a nutrition scientist, on whether it would be safe to ask men and women of any age and fitness to follow an eating plan based on 1200 calories a day for the first two weeks and then 1400 calories for the next two weeks. She confirmed it would be perfectly healthy for them to do so, providing they ate a well-balanced diet, took a multivitamin supplement and stayed properly hydrated, so I set about creating this two-stage plan.

Next, I appeared on BBC Radio Leicester to ask for volunteers to try the diet. Radio Leicester has helped me with trials before, even as far back as 1986 for my original Hip and Thigh Diet, and the listeners are really supportive. Radio presenter Tony Wadsworth is a great guy and his wife Julie Mayer, who is a roving reporter for Radio Leicester, is a real fitness fan. During the four-week trial, she held several radio interviews with some of the slimmers who described their progress on the diet. It made the whole experience great fun.

In selecting my volunteers I wanted people who, ideally, were 'virgin' dieters so that I could get as accurate a result as possible. 'Serial' dieters usually come with their own views of what works and what doesn't and would have been less likely to stick with the trial for the full four weeks. I also wanted my trial dieters to be committed to exercising almost every day. Serial dieters are notoriously not keen on exercise.

Fifty folk – both men and women – were chosen from the applications I received and their ages ranged from 18 to 70 years, with the average age being 48 years. Their weights ranged from 10st 5lb to 22st 1lb, and the average weight was 15st 6lb. We also filmed the trial dieters at the beginning of the trial and at three-monthly intervals. If you visit www.rosemaryconley.tv you will see how they transformed themselves into confident, happy, trim and healthy people. It was the first time we'd ever filmed any of our trialists because we hadn't, on previous occasions, had the opportunity to meet them in person or the facility to actually record them on film. I'm so glad we did as, when the trial dieters watch themselves on www.rosemaryconley.tv, they cannot believe what they are seeing! They had forgotten how big they once were and are so proud with themselves now that they've lost even more weight.

Each volunteer was given the option of following either the high-protein or the high-carbohydrate meal options and we ended up with 25 slimmers in each category. Interestingly, the average weight loss of each group turned out to be identical – 1 stone in the four weeks of the trial!

The greatest weight loss in 28 days was seen by 63-year-old Bill Wiltshire, who shed an astonishing 1st 10lb – the most I have ever known anyone to lose in a month! Bill started off at 22st 1lb and, four weeks later, weighed in at 20st 5lb, plus he lost 23 inches in total from his body, including five inches from his waist.

Twenty-one-year-old Ryan Flack lost 1st 9lb, reducing his weight from 21st 12lb to 20st 3lb and his body fat percentage by almost five per cent – an extraordinary achievement in just four weeks.

Our top female slimmer on the trial was 18-year-old Jane Gillespie, who slimmed down from 11st 5lb to 9st 12lb and dropped two dress sizes in four weeks!

The trial dieters came to our head office at Quorn House each week to be weighed and measured by two members of my staff – Bridget Key, who used to be a franchisee for our Clubs but now works at head office as part of our Franchise support team, and Sue White, whom I appointed as my researcher for the trial. The dieters were weighed on our special, and rather sophisticated, scales, which also measure body fat percentage. In addition to calculating each person's body mass index (BMI) and basal metabolic rate (BMR), these scales also predicted their 'metabolic age' based on all the information given and the readings taken.

When trial dieter Andy Corbett first weighed in, his metabolic age was calculated at 55 years – 10 years older than Andy's actual age of 45. After four weeks on the diet, Andy lost an amazing 1st 8lb (slimming from 15st 12lb to 14st 5lb), and his metabolic age reduced by 15 years, from 55 to 40!

Andy decided that he would rather exercise early in the day, so at six o'clock each morning he worked out to one of my DVDs. He told me that he and his wife had never laughed so much as he initially struggled with his co-ordination and felt his flab wobbling about as he exercised. After a month, he admitted that the workouts were no longer as entertaining and his wife didn't laugh as much because he could execute the routines much better now that his beer-belly and man-boobs had almost disappeared! Andy lost four inches from his waist in the four weeks.

Mark Clayton slimmed down from 16st 1lb to 14st 11lb, losing a total of 1st 4lb. Mark is 45 years old, but when he started the diet his predicted metabolic age was 60. After just four weeks his metabolic age had gone down to 38 years!

The lowest weight loss achieved over the four-week period was 8lb and there were several people who lost 11, 12 or 13lb, which was still excellent, and they were delighted with their results. Deana Merry lost 12lb, even though she went on holiday to France during the trial. And Sue Vickers admitted that she hadn't stuck rigidly to the diet but nevertheless lost 8lb and 16¾ inches in four weeks.

As we get older, our metabolic rate reduces, so I expected that my older trial dieters would not achieve anything like the average 1-stone weight loss over the four weeks, but six out of the eleven over-60s did lose a stone or more.

On the final weighing in day, the atmosphere was electric. Everyone seemed so upbeat and all the members of the trial team looked notably slimmer. The room was buzzing with stories of how their doctors had reduced their blood pressure tablets or diabetes medication and how the pains in their knees, hips, ankles had diminished! They all felt *so* much healthier and couldn't believe how quickly they had become accustomed to eating less than before and yet they hadn't gone hungry. They had enjoyed exercising and being part of the trial and were very grateful for the chance to improve their health. Dave Goodman, who lost 1st 5lb, explained to me that he'd had a fairly serious chest complaint but, after losing his excess weight, he hadn't had to use his inhaler for three weeks!

To top it all, over the four-week period the trial dieters had achieved an **average weight loss of 14lb** and lost an **average of 13.3 inches from their bodies**. I was thrilled and I felt confident that anyone else who followed the diet in this book, with all its motivational messages, daily exercise recommendations and menu suggestions at their fingertips, really could lose a stone in a month, and I was happy to make this claim.

Here are some additional comments from members of the trial team:

'This was my first diet and I can't believe how easy it was to follow and that I lost 1st 9lb in the first month! I am amazed!'
Ryan Flack (lost 1st 9lb)

'This is the easiest diet I have ever known. I can't believe the results after just four weeks. I don't feel so sleepy, my skin is much clearer and I feel much more confident. It has certainly changed my life and the way I think and feel about food. I am now well on the way to a new me!'
Helen McLeod (lost 10lb)

'I really didn't believe I could eat so much food and lose weight, but it works. I don't want this good feeling to end! My health has improved, my self-esteem is returning, I feel feminine again. I actually went in to a shop and bought a new dress and it fitted! I was so excited.'
Susan Bishop (lost 13lb)

'I have completely lost my beer belly and man boobs. Brilliant! I have really enjoyed the trial. I work out to the DVD every morning for 30 minutes. My wife says I've lost my stomach and I've stopped snoring at night. I sleep better, feel better and am generally much happier. My get up and go has come back and I feel so fit! The other morning I was walking around a park and I hadn't noticed my shorts were falling down, showing my summer-patterned underpants. This is the fashion for teenagers, not a 46-year-old!'
Andy Corbett (lost 1st 6lb)

'This was my first ever diet and I am amazed at the results. It is so easy to follow, tasted great and I didn't feel I was missing out. I am really pleased that my cholesterol has also significantly reduced.'
Mark Clayton (lost 1st 4lb)

'I feel so much healthier, and my confidence has gone sky high! My hubby thinks I'm up to no good because I'm wearing nice clothes and looking in the mirror more!'
Deana Merry (lost 12lb)

'Wow! I was absolutely thrilled. I lost 16¾ inches in total in only four weeks – including four inches from my waist. Thank you! It has really made a difference to my life.'
Sue Vickers (lost 8lb)

'Great diet. Really simple and effective and it retrained your brain and stomach to each much smaller portions without you even realising it. And it works!'
Teresa O'Neill (lost 11lb)

'I have enjoyed this diet and have never achieved such a good result on any other diet.'
Louise Slingsby (lost 1st)

'Before this diet I was under the illusion that, because of my age [60], it would be almost impossible to lose any weight. You have proved me wrong. Thank you!'
Leslie Charles (lost 10lb)

'Thank you for letting me be one of the lucky ones. I really enjoyed doing the trial and will be carrying on doing it now my mind is in the zone and I have seen such great results. The diet was easy to follow and I didn't miss anything really.'
Polly Gray (lost 10lb)

'I lost almost a stone in four weeks, but the biggest shock was my inch loss! I no longer suffer from heartburn or acid indigestion. I have more energy and can walk without getting out of breath. I can't believe how much food you can eat in one day!'
Jeanette Hopkins (lost 13.5lb)

'I felt such jubilation at losing a stone. Now I need to move forward and lose more – the best of the rest of my life is just around the corner!'
Julie Neville (lost 1st 1lb)

Six months on . . .

Several of the trial dieters have stayed in touch and come in for regular weigh-ins with Sue White and we're delighted to see that they have continued to lose weight. In the summer of

2010 we decided to run the Solo Slim diet trial along similar lines and the results were equally impressive. We have filmed several of the dieters and they too will appear on www.rosemaryconley.tv by the time this book is published.

Here are case histories of eight of the original volunteers from the trial team who succeeded in achieving results beyond their wildest dreams. I hope the tales of their individual weight-loss journeys will help motivate you to give this Amazing Inch Loss Plan your all and spur you on to ultimate slimming success.

TERESA O'NEILL
Age **36**
Height **5ft 9in (1.75m)**
Old weight **12st 9lb (80.3kg)**
New weight **11st 5½lb (72.3kg)**
Lost **1st 3½lb (8kg)**
BMI was **26.1** now **23.6**

Teresa O'Neill went from a size 16 to a size 12 in a month to fit into her dream wedding dress after taking part in the diet trial for my Amazing Inch Loss Plan.

Teresa O'Neill had the perfect motivation to lose weight – she was desperate to fit into the wedding dress she'd bought in the sales. She explains: 'I'd bought too small a dress because I thought I'd lose weight. I did try to diet a few times after buying it, but I always got side-tracked.'

Two years of an unstructured diet and hardly any exercise had turned Teresa from a fit and healthy gym bunny into an overweight bride-to-be. She admits: 'I put on weight because I stopped exercising. I just got out of the habit of going to the gym, and the weight crept on over two years. At my biggest I felt really fat. I didn't go out a huge amount but on the occasions I did, I'd try on an outfit and feel awful. I felt everything looked terrible on me.'

Unfortunately, at the same time as getting out of her good exercise habit, Teresa got into bad eating habits: 'I was eating much larger portions and my weakness was finishing off the children's tea. I didn't gorge on chips or anything, but you don't realise how many calories you're eating in normal meals.'

Weighing 12st 9lb and daunted at the prospect of her approaching wedding, Teresa applied to be a trial dieter on my Amazing Inch Loss Plan. To her relief, she was accepted on the trial and chose to follow the high-carbohydrate option. She confesses: 'It was hard at first – I wasn't used to weighing out food – but the Portion Pots® helped a lot and after the first week it felt completely normal.'

Teresa started on the 14-Day Fast Track at a challenging time as she'd booked to go on a camping holiday with friends. She recalls: 'I found it difficult to stick to the no-alcohol rule for the first two weeks because I was the only one out of our friends who stayed sober on holiday. Once we'd set up camp, a Rosemary Conley van pulled up alongside us and I thought I was being watched. It turned out to be a franchisee on holiday but it meant I was extra good.'

Teresa quickly started to feel better about herself and realised how the small sacrifices were all worth it: 'I felt like I had a big halo on my head because while I was cooking veggie chilli the others were all stuffing their faces with barbecued food and burgers. And although I now have a gin and slimline tonic at the weekend, I think avoiding alcohol during the first two weeks made a real difference.'

'I was gobsmacked at how quickly I lost the weight'
Teresa lost 11lb in the first four weeks of the diet and by the

time of her final wedding dress fitting she'd lost a total of 1st 1lb. She says: 'I felt fantastic – I was amazed that I went down two dress sizes and I could fit into all of my old clothes. More importantly, I could fit into my wedding dress! I was gobsmacked at how quickly I lost the weight.'

In August 2009, Teresa proudly walked down the aisle in her size 12 wedding dress. She recalls: 'It was a fantastic day and on my honeymoon in Greece I even wore a bikini.'

Teresa has also seen an improvement in her health: 'I'd always suffered with heartburn, but as soon as I started the diet it completely stopped. That's one of the reasons why I'm so determined to stay on the diet, it's made such a difference.'

Since her wedding day, Teresa has lost another 2.5lb, taking her total weight loss to 1st 3½lb. She has kept up her new low-fat way of eating and avoids her old habit of tucking into a takeaway curry at the weekend: 'I've bought a nice curry cookbook and I cook everything from scratch. My tikka masala tastes just as good as the takeaway. I use yogurt instead of cream and mine doesn't have all that oil on top that you get in takeaways. The whole family eat what I eat and I'm more conscious of the food we have.'

Exercise has also become a big part of Teresa's life. After getting back into gym classes, Teresa believes it's one of the main things that contributed to her weight loss. She says: 'Before the wedding, I hit the gym big time and started to enjoy exercise because it made a huge difference to my weight loss and toned up all of the flabby bits. The weight just fell off because I went to at least three gym classes a week – I find treadmills quite boring and the classes feel like a social event as well as exercise.'

Teresa now has a healthy BMI of 23.6 and feels like an entirely new person: 'I can't believe I didn't do it before because it's so easy! I feel more confident, I have more get up and go and generally feel happier.'

ANDREW CORBETT
Age **45**
Height **6ft (1.83m)**
Old weight **15st 12lb (100.7kg)**
New weight **12st 11lb (81.2kg)**
Lost **3st 1lb (19.5kg)**
BMI was **30.1** now **24.7**

A love of junk food had sent Andrew Corbett's waistline ballooning and his cholesterol and blood pressure soaring. After changing his diet and exercise habits he lost over 3 stone in six months and regained his fitness.

Cricket captain Andrew Corbett had been caught in the classic trap of denial. At his biggest, 15st 12lb, he didn't think he was overweight at all: 'I was getting more comments from my family and also the guys at work but I thought I looked fine. It wasn't until I was getting chest pains that I went to the doctor and realised it was a problem.'

Andrew discovered he had extremely high cholesterol of 7.1 as well as a high blood-pressure reading of 170/90 and his doctor immediately put him on medication. But Andrew realised he also needed to take responsibility for his own health: 'My legs were clamping up from the medication and I didn't feel good at all. As captain of the second team at my local cricket club I didn't think it looked good.'

Andrew's weight had increased steadily over the years and, with 12-hour work shifts, his diet was all over the place. He admits: 'Through the day, I'd eat sandwiches, cheese, cakes, sausage rolls, pork pies, everything. Cake was my weakness, especially fruit, date, Bakewell, lemon drizzle cakes and upside-down-puddings. I'd eat cake every day – big lumps of it. My wife Debs is really good at making them.'

But it wasn't just his working day that was a disaster for his diet. As manager of a local children's cricket team, Andrew didn't have much time at home so often chose the quick option when it came to meals: 'We ate takeaways twice a month and then I had a weakness for kebabs which I also had twice a month, along with five packets of pork scratchings a week.'

In an effort to cover his growing waistline, Andrew wore oversized T-shirts and avoided getting changed in front of his team-mates at the cricket club: 'When I played cricket my clothes fitted me like tents – big enough to hide my belly. In my cricket vest I looked like Daffyd from *Little Britain* and the lads used to do impressions of me. I was so embarrassed that I'd get changed quickly in the changing rooms so that the others wouldn't see me.'

Out on the cricket pitch Andrew struggled to keep up with all the action. He says: 'I couldn't even run between the cricket stumps.' But it wasn't only out on the cricket pitch that Andrew couldn't summon up enough energy – his lack of exercise in other areas of his life contributed to the slump in his fitness levels: 'I used to go everywhere in the car – I was lazy and lethargic and just couldn't be bothered. I couldn't run, I couldn't wear nice clothes – I couldn't even fit into extra-large sportswear.'

Andrew's wife Debs suffered many a restless night due to his size. 'My wife said I was a nightmare. I used to snore a lot – it was so bad I woke myself up. Debs told me that when I turned over in bed, she felt like a pea on a drum because I bounced the mattress so much.'

'I had hit my mid-40s and I was on a slippery slope'

In the nick of time, Andrew heard about my new diet trial and applied straight away. As strokes run in Andrew's family, a new, healthy lifestyle couldn't come soon enough: 'I had hit my mid-40s and I was on a slippery slope, as I weighed over 15st.' As if that wasn't enough to shock Andrew into action, after his 20th wedding anniversary trip to Barcelona, the photos made him realise how big he had become. He says: 'I saw the pictures of myself and knew I had to do something. They made such an impression on me that I still have one of the photos as a screensaver on my phone – just to remember what I used to look like.'

Andrew was accepted as a trial dieter and chose to follow the high-carbohydrate option. 'No alcohol for the first two weeks sounded scary at first,' he admits. 'For years, I hadn't gone without alcohol for more than two days – after a cricket match, it's very sociable and I'd always have a drink. But my fears about the diet were unfounded. It wasn't hard at all.'

As well as adapting to no alcohol for two weeks, Andrew had to get used to a whole new way of eating, after being on a cake and pastry diet for years: 'I missed the taste of kebabs at first, as well as peanuts and pork scratchings but I don't miss them now. To stick to the diet, I avoided takeaway shops completely – I didn't want the smell to tempt me.'

Andrew's taste in foods saw a complete turnaround: 'I love fruit now. Because I started the diet in the summer I ate loads of strawberries and blueberries and my taste-buds changed. I was used to tasting fat but the low-fat diet meant I could taste everything better.'

At the same time, Andrew also discovered a love of walking. After six months of recording his steps on a pedometer, he'd racked up over 1,500 miles. 'I now wear a pedometer every day to record my steps – I even work out the average number of steps that I do every week. To help keep the weight off I deliver a local community newspaper so I do loads of walking. My wife says I'm addicted to my pedometer.'

With his new eating habits and exercise regime, Andrew's weight quickly dropped off. He says: 'I was so surprised how fast I lost weight – 6lb in the first week, over a stone in a month and 2st in eight weeks. I wanted to get my BMI down to 25, but in the beginning, I thought I had no chance.'

As well as walking everywhere now, Andrew goes to classes, where he has lost another half a stone. 'If it wasn't for the trial I might never have gone to a Rosemary Conley class and danced with 40 women. But I'm so glad – the class is a community and we have such a laugh.'

'People don't recognise me'

As quickly as his weight fell off, Andrew's health improved too. He revisited his doctor after six months on the diet and the results spoke volumes. His cholesterol levels and blood pressure were perfect. He says: 'I no longer have to take tablets and I only have to see the doctor once a year, instead of once every two months.'

Andrew, who's now 47, also saw a massive difference in his appearance and it didn't go unnoticed. 'Everyone could see the difference. I had to buy new suits for cricket because they were falling off of me. I've now bought a slim-fit suit and that felt great. All my old clothes are gone – I've just kept one pair of baggy jeans. Since I've lost weight people don't recognise me – they have to do a double take.'

Andrew's new healthy eating and fitness regime has changed his whole lifestyle: 'I have more get up and go – I'll walk to the shops rather than drive. Before, I couldn't run between the cricket wickets but now I've been made Bowler of the Year. I also sleep better. I love getting up early and going for a walk around to the shop and I still wear my pedometer – the only time I take it off is for bed. I'm determined that I won't go back to what I was.'

JULIE POLE
Age **46**
Height **5ft 1½in (1.56m)**
Old weight **13st 3lb (84.1kg)**
New weight **10st 13lb (69.8kg)**
Lost **2st 4lb (14.3kg)**
BMI was **34.6** now **28.7**

A pregnancy shock and hectic family life saw Julie Pole's weight increase to over 13 stone. After following the Amazing Inch Loss Plan, Julie conquered her comfort-eating habit. She lost over 2 stone and dropped from a dress size 18 to a size 12.

When Julie Pole married husband Kevin she weighed 9st 7lb and was happy with her shape. She was no stranger to exercise as she was a regular gym goer for years. It was the surprise of her shock pregnancy that led to a bad diet, no exercise, and to Julie piling on the pounds, until she topped the scales at over 14 stone. She says: 'It was a shock to the system that I got pregnant at 37. I used to walk every day but then stopped all of a sudden and the weight just piled on. I ate too much during my pregnancy – I had strong cravings for liquorice so ate it all of the time, and I loved olives.'

But it wasn't just pregnancy weight that Julie carried. After giving birth, she and her family went through a traumatic time as her newborn was in a critical condition for 10 days in hospital. Baby Brennan had swallowed fluid and it was on his lungs. Julie recalls: 'Everything went downhill and when you're low you tend to eat more. It was a really tough time, I still get upset now when I think about it.'

Her comfort eating and lack of time meant Julie put on over 4st and her health and fitness was second to her baby. She says: 'You try to do your best by your baby, he had a bad time with his milk and cried continuously. I just used to grab the easiest thing for myself to eat. You put your baby first and the diet on the back burner – I didn't think about it.'

Like many new mums, Julie returned to full-time work but that only worsened her weight problem. 'With work and a new baby I had no time for myself,' she admits. 'My job was office-based and it became the norm to binge on biscuits – food is the first thing I went to for comfort.'

As her size continued to expand, Julie's confidence started to take a knock. She lost her passion for shopping and ended up wearing the same old clothes: 'I didn't like going shopping because I couldn't get into the clothes. I love shopping and love clothes but shops often don't do ranges for the larger lady. I hated having to go the next size up too.'

'The diet suited me and it encouraged me to exercise again'

When her son Brennan was seven years old, Julie decided it was time to start looking after her own health again. She managed to lose 11lb on her own, dropping down to 13st 3lb, but it was a colleague who prompted her to apply for the Amazing Inch Loss Plan diet trial. Julie was ready to embrace a healthy lifestyle again and was delighted to be accepted on the trial: 'The diet suited me and it encouraged me to exercise again.'

She quickly rediscovered a love for exercise and built walking into her everyday life. She says: 'To lose weight you need to do exercise – there's no point putting it off. So I was manic about how many steps I did a day and I kept a record of them. You always want to do extra and I was chuffed when I did more. For the first time in ages I felt good and one of my aims was to get into a bikini.'

Now Julie's son is nine years old and fitness has become a family affair. Julie says: 'Brennan prompts me to go for walks because he knows it's healthier to be slimmer. Since the diet I can now jog around the park – I started by just doing one round but I can do 10 laps. I do sit-ups on a bench in the park and I've also done the Race for Life. We go on long walks, bike rides and do Rosemary's DVDs in the winter.'

Even weigh-ins have become a family event. 'Every Thursday night we get on the scales and check each other's weight,' says Julie. 'I think a regular check on weight is a good thing. As a result my husband has lost around 2st 7lb and gone from an extra large clothing size to a medium. He's eating what I'm eating, he's active and he goes for bike rides with our son.'

Julie adapted the diet to suit her cravings and swapped her high-sugar, high-fat snacks for low-fat ones. 'The only thing I found difficult was cutting out olives but now I don't eat them because they're so high in fat. I started to put balsamic vinegar on salads or finely chop apricots into my food. I found healthy food that I enjoyed and drank more water. My husband Kevin cooks up slimmer soups in the winter and when I get peckish in the evening I always have strawberries or blueberries ready. I've cut out the fat in my diet and that makes a big difference.'

'It felt great getting into a size 12'

After losing 2st 4lb and dropping four dress sizes Julie has rediscovered her passion for shopping: 'It felt great getting into a size 12. The trendy shops do clothes smaller so at least I know they'll fit now. My husband loves it because he knows I feel better and my confidence has built up.'

Julie feels so good that she has braved wearing a bikini at a recent holiday to Zante in Greece. 'I took eight bikinis with me on holiday so I wore a different one every day – it was great. That was fabulous, just getting into a bikini made me feel good and now I want to get even thinner for my next holiday.'

Her new healthy lifestyle has seen her drop from a size 18 to a 12 and losing 2st 4lb has meant she can now be more active with her son. 'I was really eager to lose weight,' Julie says. 'The Amazing Inch Loss Plan was the push I needed. It encouraged me to exercise and I think that is vital.'

Julie is determined to stick to her new healthy way of life – for herself and her family. She says: 'I highly recommend the diet, it makes you feel good about yourself. The diet has changed the life of not only myself but my family too.'

RYAN FLACK
Age **21**
Height **5ft 10in (1.78m)**
Old weight **21st 12lb (138.8kg)**
New weight **18st 8lb (118kg)**
Lost **3st 4lb (20.9kg)**
BMI was **43.8** now **37.3**
Total inch loss **23.8**

Ryan Flack's weight had rocketed to nearly 22st. But moving to a new area and a new home gave him the ideal chance to break bad habits and make a fresh start. He lost 1st 9lb in just one month and more than 3 stone in six months.

Ryan Flack's bad eating habits and weight gain had affected his whole life. When he was at his heaviest – 21st 12lb – he got a lot of ribbing from his workmates. He says: 'All the lads from work used to joke about my weight. My nickname was "Bungle" and I felt like a big joke.' But, for Ryan, it was no laughing matter: 'My weight affected my work and my social life – I lost my breath just walking around.'

Old habits were hard to break, as Ryan and his workmates all tucked into a fry-up most days. He recalls: 'One fry-up was called "the heart attack" and the waitress used to give us a health warning when we ordered it. It included gammon, three sausages, five rashers of bacon, liver, steak, a few slices of fried bread, two fried eggs, a poached egg, beans, mushrooms, black pudding and buttered toast. Fry-ups were my weakness.'

'Once I lost the weight I started to feel fantastic – I'm a lot happier. I feel there's a bounce in my step as opposed to a waddle.'
Ryan Flack

When Ryan moved to Leicester from Watford in 2009, he felt it was an ideal opportunity to make some positive changes. 'I applied to be a trial dieter on Rosemary's Amazing Inch Loss Plan as I felt I needed a new start and a new me. What better time? I was in a new place and a new house.'

With an active job as a fire and security engineer, Ryan knew it was important for him to get fit. 'I travel around, fitting and fixing alarms. I really wanted to lose weight because I didn't want to be out of breath running up the stairs.'

At first, he didn't hold out too much hope about his chances of success: 'I'd never followed a diet before and I thought I wouldn't be able to. When I met the other trial dieters, I looked around and I thought I'd be the one who failed.'

But far from failing, Ryan lost an amazing 1st 9lb in just one month and was one of the top weight losers in the whole trial. Ryan admits: 'The biggest shock about the diet was how easy it was to follow. The support I had from fellow dieters made it even easier.'

'Once I lost the weight I started to feel fantastic'

After losing his excess pounds, Ryan's confidence has soared. He says: 'I thought I was happy before, when I was big, but I wasn't really. Once I lost the weight, I started to feel fantastic – I'm a lot happier. I feel there's a bounce in my step as opposed to a waddle.'

Ryan's eating habits have been transformed: 'Before I started the diet, I never felt full – it was horrible. Now I've trained myself to eat properly. If I feel hungry, I eat frozen grapes – they are tasty and last longer if they're frozen.'

Exercise has also been an important part of Ryan's weight loss: 'I've always enjoyed walking, and I've raised a lot of money for charities through completing walks. Now I've lost weight I'm hoping to walk from London to Leicester for the STEPS charity, which provides support to children with motor disorders – a charity that's dear to Rosemary's heart.'

Ryan, who's now 22, still attends my diet and fitness class in Leicester and is continuing to lose weight. He says: 'The classes are fantastic and you have a bit of a laugh. You meet people in the same position, you have the exercise and you're weighed by someone other than yourself so you're more likely to lose weight. I've also got Rosemary's *Real Results* fitness DVD and I aim to get to my target weight. The DVD is fantastic – it's good to do in between classes and it keeps you motivated. I'd advise other people to try the diet – you will prove to yourself and to other people that you can do it.'

JENNY WINNING
Age **70**
Height **5ft 4in (1.83m)**
Old weight **14st 6lb (91.6kg)**
New weight **11st 4lb (73kg)**
Lost **3st 2lb (6.8kg)**
BMI was **30.1** now **24.7**
Metabolic age was **85** now **60**

After retiring from nursing, Jenny Winning's fitness levels dropped off and the pounds piled on. But she walked her way back to fitness and lost over 3st with the help of my Amazing Inch Loss Plan.

Former nurse Jenny Winning was dismayed when her weight crept up to 14st 6lb and she could only fit into a size 18. After she'd retired from her job as a sister of cardiology she'd found herself stuck in a rut and it was a lack of exercise that had led to her weight gain. A knee injury added to the problem and the result was that her fitness levels slumped to an all-time low. She recalls: 'When I stopped work, there wasn't any motivation for me to get out and walk. As a former nurse I knew all of the risks of being overweight but it just wasn't a problem when I was working. Retiring meant a big change in my lifestyle, though, and that's when I put the weight on. Plus, my knee injury meant I couldn't play tennis any more.'

Jenny hated being overweight and became increasingly unhappy with her appearance: 'I'm not particularly tall and, when I went out, I didn't feel I looked good. I hated looking in the mirror and seeing a great big lump.'

Jenny's husband Reg, who has always been slim, also started to worry about the size of her waistline. 'My husband has always been supportive but it didn't feel good when I knew he was worried.'

So when Jenny spotted a leaflet advertising my diet trial, she realised it was just the motivation she needed: 'I wanted to lose weight but I didn't know where to start,' Jenny admits, 'I'd never been as fat as I was – so I filled in the application form the same day.'

Jenny was surprised when she heard she'd been accepted on the diet trial: 'I didn't think they'd accept me – at 70, I thought I was too old. But it made me even more determined to stick to the plan, and it's turned out to be the best thing I've ever done.'

Despite Jenny's age, her weight loss was far from slow and she lost 13¾lb in the first month and then 3st 2lb after six months. She says: 'I think you need to be much more motivated when you're older. By the age of 70, most people have retired from work and that's when you tend to put on weight. But if you stick to this diet and exercise plan you can lose weight quickly.'

It wasn't just pounds that Jenny lost, but inches too – 46¼ in total – shrinking from a size 18 to a size 12: 'It's a tremendous amount. The inches are just as important as the weight because it makes you feel better about yourself and your clothes.'

'I thought the diet was going to be hard but it was easy'
Jenny has always loved eating fruit and veg, but her habit of nibbling between meals had contributed to her growing waistline. 'I'm a nibbler and I would be again given half the chance! My weaknesses were bread, cheese, biscuits and anything savoury. I was a fussy biscuit eater – my next-door neighbour always offered me biscuits but I'd only ever have

one if they were chocolate. Evenings were also my downside –
I'd just nibble.'

But the structure of the Amazing Inch Loss Plan diet quickly
saw Jenny change her nibbling ways and she took to her new
healthy eating plan with relative ease.

'The discipline of eating three meals a day was good for
me because I'd often skipped breakfast before. I thought the
diet was going to be hard but it was easy to follow and I never
felt hungry.

'I stopped eating bread initially and now I only eat it as a
treat. Even when I went on a cruise earlier this year I didn't put
on weight, because I didn't over-indulge too much.'

Now Jenny keeps herself busy in the evenings by knitting
baby clothes. 'I keep my hands busy so I don't nibble, and that
seems to work. I also bought a good frying pan so that I don't
need to use fat or oil when I'm cooking.'

After the first month on the diet Jenny had worried that
her motivation levels might waver. But her husband Reg came
to the rescue with the aid of household bricks. 'Reg built a
small wall in our garden and, as I lost weight he removed one
brick at a time. Now when I see overweight people, I can
visualise how many extra bricks they're carrying in weight. It
was a great motivation because you can see how much you're
losing. Each brick weighs 2lb so they're a good tool.'

Jenny has now adapted the diet to suit their lifestyle, and
they eat their main meal at midday instead of the evening.
She explains: 'I have more time in the day so it makes sense to
have our main meal then. Once you're retired it's possible to
do this and it works better for us.'

Jenny has also been careful to maintain a social life and
when she goes to friends for dinner she still enjoys herself. 'I
wouldn't refuse food at a friend's house but now they know

I'm dieting they are very supportive and cook low-fat things for me. They prepare healthier dinners and I have a smaller portion, making sure I fill up with veg.'

'It's exercise that really makes the difference'

After starting the diet Jenny began to walk everywhere and she quickly saw improvements to her health. 'At first I was out of breath and slow because I was unfit and obese. My knee was painful but now it's a lot better.'

The Rosemary Conley pedometer was a big motivator for Jenny, and she usually achieves well over the recommended 10,000 steps a day. 'I couldn't walk 10,000 steps a day at first but now I walk every day – and I have a following of other people who join me for walks. They've seen the results are great and how it's improved my life. If I can't walk, I'll work out to a fitness DVD instead, but we walk in all weathers – that shows true motivation.'

'I was a size 18 when I started, I can now get into size 12 jeans.'
Jenny Winning

Walking was a great option for Jenny because she didn't feel comfortable with the idea of going to a gym or fitness club. 'With age, things tend to drop and you can become flabby. You're loathe to join a gym, because you feel it will be full of young people. But walking is the ultimate answer because it's the exercise that really makes a difference.'

Jenny, who's now 71, still wants to lose another 9lb to reach her dream weight. 'I was a size 18 when I started. I can now get into size 12 jeans, but I'd like to feel a bit more comfortable in them.' And she has plenty of motivation to lose those final pounds.

Jenny's husband is delighted with her weight loss and other people have noticed the difference in her. 'Reg is really pleased – he thinks I look good now. I *feel* good now and lots of people have complimented me on my weight loss. People tell me I'm looking good and that makes me feel great.'

As well as losing weight, Jenny has become fitter. She says: 'My knee no longer hurts and I'm even going to see if I can play tennis again later this year. The plan has taught me that I can have the odd indulgence but I know what to do to get back on track. I'm so thankful for the diet trial – it gave me the motivation I needed. If I can stick to it – anyone can.'

JANE GILLESPIE
Age **18**
Height **5ft 1in (1.55m)**
Old weight **11st 5lb (72.1kg)**
New weight **8st 9lb (54.9kg)**
Lost **2st 10lb (17.2kg)**

A diet of fast food and chocolate saw teenager Jane Gillespie's waistline expand. But after losing 2st 10lb in six months, Jane has binned her junk-food habit for good.

Eighteen-year-old Jane Gillespie was the youngest of our trial team. She lost 1st 7lb and trimmed 13½ inches off her figure, slimming down from 11st 5lb to 9st 12lb in just one month. Since then, Jane has gone on to lose more weight.

As an overweight spotty teenager, Jane had never worried about the mounds of unhealthy processed food she was eating. At just over 5ft tall, she weighed 11st 5lb and squeezed into size 14 clothes. She admits: 'I've always been a big girl, but over the years you don't realise how big you are getting.'

During her teens, Jane had stuck to food that was easy to make and turned down meals her mum cooked. She says: 'If I didn't like what my mum offered I'd cook my own dinner – normally something frozen and with chips.'

She often skipped breakfast and would snack on unhealthy food through the day to satisfy her hunger pangs. 'I ate all the bad stuff whether it was chocolate or fast food – I didn't worry about my diet at the time.'

In Jane's world of quick-fix food it didn't occur to her that her weight might be a problem as she fuelled her body with unhealthy, stodgy meals: 'I'd eat chocolate every day and a McDonald's once a week, as well as big dinners with chips. I didn't eat much veg because I didn't think I needed to.'

Jane admits now that her confidence suffered: 'When I put on clothes, I didn't think I looked nice but I just put it to the back of my mind. I was in denial because I didn't want to admit that I was big. I also used to get really big spots and I think that was down to my unhealthy diet.'

And Jane might have continued with her unhealthy eating habits were it not for the intervention of her grandma, who had wanted to apply for the Amazing Inch Loss Plan diet trials herself, but instead filled the form in for Jane. Initially, Jane had her doubts. 'I'd tried other diets, but I never succeeded in losing weight. Applying to be a trial dieter was quite scary because I didn't know what to expect.'

But, after being accepted on the trials, Jane's worries soon cleared. 'It took a couple of weeks to adapt but in the end I found the diet easy – the weight was disappearing fast.'

It wasn't until Jane started to lose inches that it struck her how overweight she'd become during her teenage years. 'I didn't look at myself and think I was fat. I only realised how big I was when I looked at photos of myself when I was younger and compared them to my teen pictures – I was big.'

'I never felt hungry on the diet'

For Jane, starting the Amazing Inch Loss Plan diet meant swapping frozen junk food for fresh, healthy food. 'The first couple of weeks were hard but I soon got used to eating veg and I couldn't believe how much bad stuff I ate before.'

The diet taught Jane to eat more regularly and to control her portion sizes and she no longer suffered from hunger pangs. She says: 'When I was bigger I used to eat big portions, but not very often. I'd skip breakfast and then have a big lunch and dinner because I was constantly hungry. But when I started the diet it felt like I was eating all of the time – I was never hungry. I also started to drink more water and I think that helped to fill me up too.'

'Seeing how much weight you've lost keeps you motivated.'
Jane Gillespie

Jane also discovered a love of exercising, especially cycling. 'I love riding my bike and on a trip to Center Parcs we rode our bikes all day – I would never have been able to do that before.'

In the past Jane had always shunned exercise and would feel embarrassed if she got out of breath. 'I avoided exercise because I didn't want to get upset if I couldn't do it. I was worried I'd get left behind if we were cycling together. I'm much fitter now, I don't get out of breath walking and I can run to work and back.'

As well as seeing an improvement in her fitness levels, Jane has also seen a difference in her skin: 'My skin is a lot better now. I used to get spots, but now it's clear – I think it's down to eating lots of green veg – it's helped a lot.'

Jane's now in her twenties and her weight is as healthy as her diet. Her new looks have not gone unnoticed as she's shrunk from a size 14 to a size 8/10. 'I feel great. Everyone looks at me now and they can't believe how good I look. I had to chuck loads of my clothes away.'

Jane has come a long way since her frozen dinner days: 'The diet is my life now – the healthy food I eat is what I'll always have. It's not just about how fat I was – eating how I used to eat is ridiculous and unhealthy – I don't even have to think about it now.'

Jane has stayed motivated the whole way through the diet, and the quick results with her weight loss proved to be a big help: 'I got so much support on the diet and the encouragement of looking at the scales and seeing how much weight you've lost keeps you motivated. Everyone should try it – this is the best diet ever.'

JEANETTE HOPKINS
AGE **36**
Height **5ft 4in (1.63m)**
Old weight **12st 6lb (78.9kg)**
New weight **10st 1lb (64kg)**
Lost **2st 5lb (14.9kg)**
BMI was **29.7** now **24.1**
Total inch loss **32½in**

Jeanette Hopkins was shocked into action after seeing holiday snaps of herself. She lost 2st 5lb and dropped from a size 14/16 to a size 10 in six months on my Amazing Inch Loss Plan.

Jeanette Hopkins had gained her excess pounds steadily over 10 years until she topped the scales at 12st 6lb. But it wasn't until she saw the photos her daughter had taken of her on an Egyptian holiday that she realised how much she had ballooned.

She says: 'I didn't bother with mirrors when I was big. After seeing the holiday photos, I felt ashamed and embarrassed at how big I'd become and I knew I had to do something, I had to change. Being overweight is horrible – it knocks your confidence.'

Jeanette's self-esteem had taken a battering, but her health suffered, too. She recalls: 'I couldn't walk far and I was always out of breath. I was a couch potato. I was living the lazy lifestyle and I had no energy. The worst thing was my severe heartburn. I couldn't go anywhere without taking tablets, it was that bad.'

But it wasn't just Jeanette's lazy lifestyle that caused her weight to rocket; her diet had played a big part, too. Addicted to coffee and sugar, Jeanette would go for hours without food and then binge on fatty foods. She admits: 'I have an addictive nature and when things are taken away from me I want them more. I used to skip breakfast and not have much to eat at lunch but then I pigged out at dinner and in the evening. I used to have four or five vodkas every evening and then, when I felt tipsy, I ate more. I ate too much food and it was the wrong food. Everything was cooked in olive oil and my weaknesses were Sunday roasts and chocolate.'

'The diet and the daily activities are brilliant. If you haven't got much time, there are some really quick solutions to exercise.'
Jeanette Hopkins

Just two days after Jeanette returned from her Egyptian holiday, still in shock over her size, her husband heard me on the radio appealing for trial dieters. Jeanette felt she fitted the bill so she applied to take part in the trial.

Jeanette was relieved when she was accepted and she chose the high-protein option on the diet. She says: 'I went straight to the supermarket to buy everything I needed for the week. At first, it was a bit difficult for my mind to adjust. It was a hard decision to start the diet but I knew I couldn't go on the size I was.'

In the end, the diet wasn't as hard to follow as Jeanette had first thought: 'I can't believe how much I'm allowed to eat, I can stick to the diet easily. The diet and the daily activities are brilliant. If you haven't got much time, there are some really quick solutions to exercise.'

'My husband doesn't believe I'm the same woman'

Amazingly, Jeanette lost 13lb in the first four weeks of the diet and wanted to be certain that her weight loss continued. She says: 'I didn't want the diet to be a quick fix. I knew I'd lost weight fast but I wanted to carry on and remain focused. I joined Rosemary's class to make sure I did the exercise but now the classes keep me going, so I don't slip into bad habits. I've made so many friends – it's fantastic being able to share achievements with everyone else. One lady told me I was an inspiration to her because she'd seen the transformation in me.'

Jeanette now looks stunning and her confidence has soared. She says: 'My husband doesn't believe I'm the same woman – he feels like he's having an affair with someone else! Before I lost weight I didn't even like going out with my husband – I felt I was an embarrassment. But now I feel so much better about myself.'

Now that Jeanette has lost nearly 2½ stone, her health has benefited hugely. She no longer suffers from heartburn and walks more than eight miles every Sunday without getting out of breath: 'My health improvements are literally all down to the diet. I now love walking, I go to Rosemary's class every Monday and I exercise to DVDs at home. I'm amazed at myself – I've been converted to the Rosemary Conley way and it's so easy.'

Jeanette lost inches as well as weight – she shed 32½ inches in just six months. She admits: 'I still automatically pick up a size 14 when I go shopping, just out of habit. But I'm now trying on size 10s. I used to buy a size 14 without trying it on and then I'd squeeze into the clothes.'

The diet has also had a positive impact on Jeanette's family. She says: 'My daughter has started eating the same food as me. Before, she wouldn't touch it but she's tried some of the recipes I've made and doesn't even realise they're low fat. I am honoured to have been selected for the diet trial and will be eternally grateful to Rosemary for turning my life around.'

Jeanette has now become something of a celebrity herself as she was selected as the successful slimmer to appear on three million Rosemary Conley Diet and Fitness Club leaflets and posters for Rosemary's Easter advertising campaign in 2010, and she has also featured in several women's national magazines.

POLLY GRAY
Age **60**
Height **5ft 2in (1.57m)**
Old weight **11st 1lb (70.1kg)**
New weight **8st 11lb (55.6kg)**
Lost **2st 4lb (14.5kg)**
BMI was **35.1** now **22.3**
Metabolic age was **63** now **46**
Total inch loss **29.5**

Polly Gray has a new-found confidence and a new attitude to food after losing 2st 4lb in six months on my Amazing Inch Loss Plan.

After years of letting the pounds creep on, Polly Gray has transformed her body and can finally wear the clothes she wants since losing her excess pounds and dropping from a dress size 14/16 to an enviable size 10.

At her heaviest, Polly had topped the scales at 11st 1lb and she knew she had to make some changes to her diet. She admits: 'The weight just crept on over the years. I was eating the wrong things but I didn't necessarily think it was wrong.'

As soon as she heard my plea on BBC Radio Leicester for trialists for my Amazing Inch Loss Plan, Polly realised that this was a chance to finally do something about her weight and she quickly got in touch. She says: 'I thought it would be a fantastic opportunity. I knew that if you have help when dieting it makes it much easier. I was so lucky to be chosen, I just had to change.'

As the weight piled on over the years, Polly had suffered from low self-esteem: 'I was fat, ugly and uncomfortable. I didn't wear the clothes that I wanted to because I didn't feel good. But now I was ready to lose weight and I knew I'd put 100 per cent effort into it.'

Although Polly had always enjoyed fresh fruit and vegetables, she realises now that it was eating too many carbohydrates that had caused her weight to soar. 'I was terrible, when I made sandwiches I would layer the butter on, and I was also a bit of a naughty cake eater. Most of all I was a potato freak – I'd eat mashed potato and jacket potato with loads of butter and cheese, and even potato sandwiches!'

Polly's previous man-sized portions have now halved and her potato-sandwich days are long gone. She insists: 'I don't have anything like that now. Since I started the diet I've been very strict with myself.'

Polly has also got into the habit of checking labels at the supermarket and making better food choices. 'Nowadays so many products have clear fat content information on them so it's easy to choose the right foods. Before I started the diet, I didn't realise what was bad for you, but now I know you can eat perfectly well without all that fat and too many calories.'

'My energy levels are so much better'

As you'd expect, Polly chose to follow the high-carbohydrate option on the diet and in the first month she lost 10lb and quickly started to notice the difference in her health and fitness. She says: 'I've always gone walking on a Sunday with my girlfriends and I used to lag behind and question whether we had to walk that far. But now my energy levels are so much better I'm the one at the front telling everyone else to stop lagging behind. I also notice a difference when I go to the gym, I feel so much better. Once it gets into your blood you want to do more exercise – you feel the benefits straight away.'

Now that Polly is so close to her goal weight she's feeling better than ever: 'I don't want to sound like I'm blowing my own trumpet but I look at myself and think, "you're looking OK girl".'

Polly, now 61, looks more than 'OK', she looks stunning and beams with confidence. 'I look at myself in a different light and I can now wear what I want.'

Healthy eating has not only benefited Polly but her family too, and her twin sons have both lost weight. 'We've had nothing naughty in the house and I've cut their portion sizes. They joked about the diet at first but now they're just pleased they've lost weight.'

There's no stopping Polly now and she's determined to stick with her new healthy eating habits. She says: 'Once you start seeing the results you'll want to carry on. The diet is easy to follow and there's a variety of food – you've got to give it a go. We are all thrilled with the results. It can change your life and how you feel about yourself.'

3 It works! It really, really works!

When the Lord Mayor of Leicester's trousers fell down at a public engagement at a school because he'd lost weight on my diet, the story hit the headlines across the world. Councillor Colin Hall's embarrassing moment was reported as far afield as CNN and ABC television networks in America and even in India! The Lord Mayor had been following my Amazing Inch Loss Plan since taking office a month earlier. At his first weigh-in, Councillor Hall had lost a stone and two month's later he'd lost another. Councillor Hall was determined to set a good example and to promote healthy eating and being more ative during his year in office and had sought my help. He walked to many of his official engagements and adopted a low-fat lifestyle. His example was inspirational.

Nora Parminter, a journalist with the *Crediton Country Courier*, tested my Amazing Inch Loss Plan diet in January 2010 and lost a stone in one month. Nora, who has a wheat and gluten intolerance, chose the high-protein options on the diet and was surprised at the variety of food she was able to eat. As well as helping her to lose weight, the diet has encouraged her into healthier eating habits.

Here's a copy of the article that Nora wrote for the *Crediton Country Courier*, in February 2010:

My D-Day has arrived!

A huge change in my personal circumstances threw me into turmoil at the end of 2009, making Christmas really tough to cope with. My stress levels went through the roof and I resorted to comfort eating.

By the time the New Year arrived I had overindulged to the extent where I was actually looking forward to starting Rosemary Conley's Amazing Inch Loss Plan and consuming some healthy food!

I was very excited about starting the 28-day diet plan and as I studied each daily menu was amazed at the choice of healthy, low-fat, low-Gi foods included in the diet. Although each day has its own menu plan, each meal is calorie counted and interchangeable, so if I do not have the right ingredients (I'm not very organised at the moment!) I can swap one meal for another in the same category.

I thought I would have problems because I have to avoid wheat and gluten, but it has encouraged me to eat fewer carbohydrates, more protein and more fruit and vegetables.

As well as the diet plan, Rosemary's people kindly sent me a Magic Measure, which is a modified tape measure with coloured markers, some of which can be attached permanently and some are temporary. With this ingenious device I was able to permanently fix the colour coded markers to the tape to record my measurements at the start of the diet, then to add temporary ones at the end of each week. This is a great motivational tool, which helps me to see how much weight I lose each week as well as how much I have lost since the beginning of the diet.

My Magic Measure is currently showing a loss of two inches from my bust, three from my waist and two from my hips and that's just in three weeks. When I spoke to Rosemary on the telephone, she was very enthusiastic about the diet and said that she had never before made the claim in any of her books that it was possible to lose a stone in a month. But I can see that it really is possible to do it and in a healthy way.

The first two weeks on the diet were tough because I was only allowed 1200 calories per day and at one point I became so hungry that, just for a fleeting moment, I considered licking my plate!

It was just my luck that as soon as I started the diet the weather changed and 'sunny Devon' became more like Antarctica! I am sure this made me feel much hungrier than I would otherwise have been. At one point I was snowed in at home all day with a fridge full of food. This required a lot of willpower and a padlock!

For the third and fourth weeks of the plan the calorie intake increases to 1400 a day and I found this much easier as I can now add a dessert and an alcoholic drink or a treat to the breakfast, morning power snack, lunch, afternoon power snack and dinner that I was previously allowed. In fact I'm probably eating more than I did before, but eating healthier food.

My weight loss at the end of week three was a lot less than in the previous two weeks and I did feel a little disheartened until I read Rosemary's motivational advice for the day and it made me feel much better.

At the end of week two, having lost 10lb I went into Exeter to meet up with a friend and every few steps I took I had to pull up my jeans and I got some very strange looks from people. In the end I bought myself another pair of jeans in a smaller size, a size I've not been able to wear for many years.

My annual blood pressure check a few days ago showed that my blood pressure had come down, which is great news. And to top it all my fourth weekly weigh-in showed that I'd lost a stone in a month! I am absolutely delighted and I'm feeling huge benefits already.

I would happily recommend this diet to anyone who wants to lose weight and improve their health and fitness levels.

Six months later, Nora updated me on her progress. She wrote:

Losing a stone at the beginning of the year made me feel fitter, happier and healthier and I am delighted to have kept the weight off by adopting a healthier way of eating.

Since my original *Amazing Inch Loss Plan* book was published I have received hundreds of letters, emails, Twitter and Facebook messages from readers and Rosemary Conley Club members who were delighted with their weight and inch losses. Many also reported increased health benefits.

Four Rosemary Conley Club members who achieved spectacularly successful results on my Amazing Inch Loss Plan were Stephanie Hughes, Michael Hutchinson, Carl Williams and Eve Leonard.

Stephanie Hughes, 35, was desperate to lose weight and get fitter and healthier so that she could be a better role model for her six-year-old daughter. Stephanie, from High Wycombe in Buckinghamshire, joined her local class on 4 January 2010, weighing 23st 8lb, and by 11 October of that year, she had lost an incredible 12st 1lb and 119 inches by following my Amazing Inch Loss Plan. She was crowned Rosemary Conley Big Loser Female Slimmer of the Year 2011.

After joining the class, Stephanie had also discovered a love of exercise, something she'd never thought possible before. She says:

I was amazed that I found the diet so easy – I haven't struggled once. I didn't crave for anything and I felt like I was eating quite a lot. I'm also amazed that I now love exercise – I couldn't say that a year ago. I have loads of energy now, I've turned into a fidget and can't keep still.

Stephanie found my Magic Measure a brilliant motivating tool in her weight loss campaign and was surprised how quickly the weight and inches came off:

> *I was shocked at how quickly I lost the weight and I'm still not used to the new me. It's the best thing I've ever done. It's been fantastic!*

Now that she has lost her excess weight, Stephanie is confident enough to start training for a career as a driving instructor – something she wouldn't have done if she was still overweight.

> *My whole mindset has changed. To feel like I have achieved something by losing weight is a new way of thinking for me.*

Twenty-six-year-old Michael Hutchinson, from Sittingbourne in Kent, joined his local Rosemary Conley class in January 2010 weighing 30st 7lb, and by October that year he had lost an astonishing 10 stone. He was crowned Rosemary Conley Big Loser Male Slimmer of the Year 2011.

Before starting the Amazing Inch Loss Plan Michael, who's a psychiatric nurse, was seriously worried about his health, and he knew his wife was too. He had considered having a gastric band fitted, but now he's determined to stick with his new healthy low-fat way of eating. He says:

> *The weight just fell off because I stuck to the diet – I couldn't believe it! The diet made a lot of sense to me and that was so important – it's so structured and easy to follow. I've been on loads of diets in the past, but this is so simple. This diet has helped me learn about myself and different foods – it's changed my life. I also*

achieved the goal of my wife not having to worry about
my weight – now I feel like a good husband.

Michael also saw a significant drop in his blood pressure as well as an improvement in his overall health:

I am feeling much healthier and I feel that my body
has become a lot more responsive to what I put into it.
My blood pressure has come down from 180/100 (at
its worse) to 117/64 (at its best), and my heart rate
has come down from around 100 bpm to 44 bpm (at
its best.) As well as the obvious health benefits, I am
feeling so much more confident than I ever have done,
which is having a really positive effect on my
relationship and the work that I do. I also don't feel
like a hypocrite when I give healthy living advice to my
patients, which I always found a problem in the past.

Thirty-eight-year-old Carl Williams, from Llangaffd in Anglesey, had always struggled with his weight. Then in 2009 he became unemployed. Nothing seemed to be going right for him and his weight soared to an unhealthy 23st 1lb. Carl realised he couldn't carry on the way he was, so he used up all of his savings to become a Premier Club member at his local Rosemary Conley class.

It turned out to be the right decision, because Carl lost 9 stone in just six months on my Amazing Inch Loss Plan and received our Rosemary Conley Super-Fit Male Slimmer of the Year 2011 award. He now has the confidence to attend job interviews and feels that no job is out of his reach:

I grabbed the diet by the horns and now I've done it I
couldn't be happier. My life has completely turned

*around. The diet has opened up so many doors for me
and now I have so much confidence. It's never too late
to lose weight. It makes such a difference to your life
and overall health.*

Student Eve Leonard, 22, from Lancaster, had piled on the
pounds while she was at university and was unhappy with her
16st 8lb weight. So when her boyfriend booked their first
holiday she decided it was time to do something about it. Eve
joined her local Rosemary Conley class and lost 5st 10lb in just
nine months on my Amazing Inch Loss Plan while studying for
a Masters degree. She received our Rosemary Conley Student
Slimmer of the Year 2011 award.

Eve was surprised how quickly she adapted to the diet and
how fast the weight came off, and healthy eating and exercise
are now part of her everyday life. She says:

*Following the calorie allowance really worked for me –
everything was controlled. The diet is easy to follow
because everything is explained well and the classes
are a great support. The diet is now part of my life –
it's changed the way I cook and eat. It encourages
healthy eating and exercise – I now believe you need
both to lose weight.*

Reader Tess Wilkins, who contacted me via Facebook, wrote:

*Thank you so much for the Amazing Inch Loss Plan! It
really, really works, and I'm so grateful. It's great to
lose inches all over, but just thought I'd mention that
it REALLY works for hips and thighs, too. I've lost six
inches from my hips and two inches from each thigh in
five months (and 23lb in weight). Shopping is now a*

LOVELY experience, rather than an embarrassing chore. Rosemary – you are wonderful!

Claire Noone lost an incredible 6st 7lb, slimming down from 21st 10lb to 15st 3lb. She also lost 10 inches off her bust, 10 inches off her waist, 10 inches off her hips, 9 inches off her widest part, 4 inches off her arms, 7 inches off her thighs and 7 inches off her knees! Claire is continuing on the plan and aiming to get down to her target weight of 10 stone.

Claire wrote:

I have been on a mission this year to finally lose the weight I've piled on over the years. I started on 4th January 2010 weighing in at 21st 10lb and currently I weigh 15st 3lb! When my children were younger I attended one of your Clubs and was successful at losing quite a bit of weight. Your ethos has stayed with me over the years and has made it easier and more enjoyable to lose the weight now. I still have about 4 stone to go, but know that I will do it. I'm told by family, friends and colleagues at work that I look like a new woman – I'm certainly feeling like one.

Jenny Carruthers loved the diet although she admitted she had not managed to sort out a regular regime. Nevertheless, she lost a stone and 17 inches and dropped a dress size in eight weeks. Jenny commented:

Overall I feel this is probably the best diet I have tried and, believe me, I have tried many! I hope to lose another stone and a half and my new goal is to be able to send you another letter to record a further stone lost by the end of the summer.

Club member Jessica Hardiment wrote to say how much she enjoyed following the plan:

> *The combination of the quick and filling meals and regular exercise has helped me to lose 17lb in the first four weeks and I have not felt deprived. Gone is the idea that I must have bread and potatoes to fill me up; the high-protein, low-carbohydrate choices leave me perfectly satisfied. Now the 14-Day Fast Track part of the diet is over and my target weight is closer, I feel confident and motivated to carry on, with a little help from my new friends in class!*

Christine Rayner, who lost a stone, wrote:

> *I have followed, together with my husband, the Amazing Inch Loss Plan for six weeks and lost a stone! Hubby has lost 1½ stone. We are so pleased and I am continuing until I have shed another 7–8lb. I dropped from size 18 to 16 in four weeks. I am absolutely thrilled with the results and we plan to stick with low-fat eating for the rest of our lives.*

Mike Walsh, 56, loves his beer and his food and his weight had crept up without his really noticing. His wife, Gill, joined a Rosemary Conley class and they encouraged each other on their weight-loss campaign and have lost almost 6 stone between them.

Mike wrote:

> *It hasn't felt like being on a diet, it's felt like rediscovering the real us. The satisfaction of knowing that I control what goes into my body is very powerful*

*and provides the positive reinforcement needed to
keep going when the scales stick.*

*The main thing – the only thing – is that the diet
works, and I have now achieved my target of getting
from nearly 15 stone to below 12 stone, of being able
to swing a golf club like I used to, of getting back into
trousers I thought I should throw away, and of not
settling for a plump and lethargic middle age. And Gill
– having recovered from breast cancer last year – looks
terrific.*

I also received many letters and messages from slimmers who
experienced substantial improvements to their health and
wellbeing. One of these was sixty-three-year-old Bob. At 5ft
9in, Bob was unhappy with his 17st 8lb weight. In 2009 he'd
been diagnosed with Type 2 diabetes and also had high blood
pressure and cholesterol readings. He was subsequently
prescribed a 12-week course at a Rosemary Conley class to
help him lose weight. This is what he wrote:

*In October 2009 I was diagnosed with Type 2
diabetes. My blood sugar was high, as was my
cholesterol level and blood pressure, and it was
explained to me that this is a serious, life-threatening
condition but that it could be managed and controlled
by drugs and a change of lifestyle.*

*Over a period of about six months and some trial
and error, the diabetic nurse arrived at a cocktail of
drugs that I could take without obvious side effects,
and this was successful in reducing my blood sugar,
cholesterol and blood pressure to more acceptable
levels. However, the drugs did nothing to make me feel
better in myself or to make it easier to achieve the*

necessary lifestyle changes. I needed to lose weight and I knew that this could only be achieved through diet and exercise.

The dietician attached to my surgery, having unsuccessfully tried a range of ways to support me, offered me a 12-week course on prescription with a slimming club, and gave me a choice of three that were running in my locality. I remember thinking, cynically, that this was the last thing that would work for me. Little did I know . . . I chose to enrol at the Rosemary Conley Club because this was the only one that offered exercise as well as a discreet weigh-in, personal advice, and guidance on lifestyle and healthy eating.

Bob wrote to me again in January 2010, after starting at the class:

My initial fears seemed to be confirmed when I arrived at my first meeting. I was one of only two men and I felt very alone and exposed; I felt that I was the odd one out and would not fit in, but I couldn't have been more wrong. Everyone was warm and welcoming and determined to make me feel comfortable and at ease, and when I met Rachel, who leads the group, my negativity just drained away. Her advice and guidance is always encouraging and supportive, emphasising what we can do as opposed to what we can't, and her sense of humour and delivery makes everything fun and enjoyable.

The acknowledgement, the knowledge and the understanding that long-term success is not achieved without occasional setbacks along the way, but that

we can overcome them, has been the key for my
achieving the life changes I've failed to achieve in the
past. This, together with the realisation that exercise
can be fun and something to be enjoyed for its own
sake, rather than simply a means to an end. I am
confident that my lifestyle has changed and that,
while the battle to maintain the changes will be
ongoing, I will continue to remain confident as long as
I am a member of the Club.

Bob wrote once more, in April 2010, to update me on his progress. His blood sugar, cholesterol, and blood pressure were now within normal limits and his diabetic nurse was monitoring his progress with a view to reducing his medication. Bob has lost 2st 5lb, down from 17st 8lb to 15st 3lb and is continuing to lose weight. He wrote:

I now exercise regularly: walking, cycling, or working
out at home doing the exercises I've learned at the
club. I follow Rosemary's advice regarding low-fat
foods and calorie counting and can honestly say I
rarely feel hungry and feel much better mentally and
physically. More importantly, I enjoy the exercise and
look forward to it.
*   I'll always be grateful to all of the people who have*
helped me to regain control.

Businesswoman Kristina Freer had been trying to get her blood pressure down for 10 years. The pounds had crept on steadily after the onset of the menopause when she started HRT and then found herself comfort-eating. At size 18, she tried several diets, including Weight Watchers, Atkins, Mayo Clinic, Cabbage Diet and even Magic Knickers! But nothing had worked, until she joined her local Rosemary Conley Club in Birstall, Leicestershire. After following my Amazing Inch Loss Plan she lost 1st 7lb in eight weeks.

Kristina wrote:

The last visit to the doctor for my six-monthly check-up saw my blood pressure drop from 160/90 to 124/64! He said if I maintained the weight loss he would consider reducing the strength of my tablets. Here's hoping. Also, I had been under the hospital for a dodgy eye for five years. As part of the procedure they also monitored the pressure in my eyes. When I attended my last appointment recently, I was discharged and the nurse who was looking after me, told me that the pressure in both my eyes had also come down to normal. I can only assume it was down to my reduced blood pressure, which was a direct result of my weight loss.

Club member Jacqui Tuckley lost 2 stone on the Amazing Inch Loss Plan and has been able to stop taking her blood pressure medication. At first, she wasn't keen on exercise but got stuck in and now works out regularly to my fitness DVDs. She wrote:

'I'm 2 stone lighter and so thrilled. I had been diagnosed with high blood pressure but have now stopped taking the tablets as it has dropped to a more acceptable level.'
Jacqui Tuckley

Here I am in May 2010, 2 stone lighter and so thrilled with myself I can't begin to tell you. I had been diagnosed with high blood pressure in December but have now stopped taking the tablets as it has dropped to a more acceptable level.

*I have bought your exercise DVDs and use them
regularly – and I even enjoy it. I continue to use my
faithful little books [member packs] because the food
is so delicious. Another advantage, which I had never
considered, is that I spend approximately £20 a week
less at the supermarket!*

*So thank you Rosemary and all your team. Your
efforts in putting together the diet and fitness regime
has really paid off for me and I will continue to follow
them.*

Club member Jackie Nathan, who's 70 years old, suffered from
high blood pressure and a kidney disorder. A marriage
proposal inspired her to tackle her weight and, in doing so, she
improved her health. She wrote:

*I met a man a few years ago that I knew would
make me happy. Last year we decided to get married.
After the service I promised to give him 30 years. As
we are both 70, that was a rash statement to make.
I decided this year to help towards that goal. I was
very overweight, I have a kidney disorder and was
very breathless and suffered from high blood
pressure.*

*After three months I am no longer breathless, I've
lost 22 inches all over, gone down two dress sizes on
my top half and one size on my bottom half and my
blood pressure is normal. This is all thanks to the
Rosemary Conley diet and my diet and fitness
instructor Susannah Wyeth who gives encouragement
all the time. I still have some way to go but know I will
get there.*

Club member Vicki Green had suffered with irritable bowel syndrome (IBS) and found that the diet helped to reduce her symptoms. She wrote:

I have suffered with irritable bowel syndrome (IBS) for 13 years. The symptoms include severe stomach cramps, bloating after EVERY meal, lethargy (when having an attack which was almost daily), severe constipation, resulting in my frequently taking laxatives, and terrible wind, which is probably the most embarrassing part of my condition. I have been prescribed lots of different medication for IBS – peppermint capsules, anti-spasmodic drugs and laxatives, all of which have helped parts of my condition but not all of them.

I went through a process of eliminating foods that bring on an attack and I have, after 13 years, discovered that I am intolerant to lots of food from mushrooms to white onions. Although I had begun to control the cramps through diet, I still suffered with wind, constant bloating and constipation and the doctors basically told me it was something I had to 'put up with'. I have also realised that if I am stressed or tired one week, the following week my IBS is really bad and it has resulted in me having to have time off work.

I stopped smoking a year and a half ago after 16 years on 10–15 cigarettes a day, as according to the experts smoking can make IBS worse. I put a stone and a half on and felt utterly miserable, but my IBS didn't improve. My friend had been attending your classes for over a year and I asked her if I could go with her. After three months of following the diet plan and fitness classes, which I love, I started to notice that I wasn't having daily attacks and that I didn't need to take laxatives three or five times a week as my body had started to respond to this new healthy lifestyle.

After six months of being a member of Rosemary Conley Clubs I can honestly and happily say that my attacks are very few and far between. The healthy diet and exercise has made me feel more confident and has helped put IBS into the background of my life. It no longer controls me, I control it.

Cholesterol

Ana-Maria Hutchinson lost 1st 12lb, and has seen a reduction in her cholesterol. She wrote:

Not only did I reach my ideal weight of 9st 4lb, I've actually lost some more and I'm now stable at 8st 7lb in the morning (probably 8st 11lb in the evening with trainers on), still a very healthy weight for my 5ft 4½in. I'm very happy with my weight and I've managed to maintain it by sticking to the diet during the week and also at weekends (using the Portion Pots®, counting the calories, eating 5% or less fat, and generally following all the dietary advice) except when I eat out, where I will indulge a bit more, but without excess.

My relationship with food has improved a lot and I don't rely on it any more for comfort. It's also true, however, that as I want to avoid putting the weight back on at all costs, I now look at food as a potential fattening agent, so I'm very cautious where food is concerned and perhaps not as relaxed as I could be when I'm supposed to be enjoying myself, like at parties.

I'd also like to report that I jogged the Cancer Research Race for Life with my daughter and a friend and raised a fabulous £700. I managed to jog practically the whole 5k – it was as if I'd been given wings! Prior to the event and the training for it, I only used to walk, never jog. I completed the 5k in under 39 minutes – several minutes ahead of my daughter, who's slim and 25 years old – and what a fantastic feeling that was! A friend took pictures of me crossing the finishing line and I have them in my bedroom, on my vision board – together with my final RC weight loss certificate – to remind me of what I can achieve!

My cholesterol level, which was 6.7 two years ago, went down to 5.5 at the beginning of this year. This is still higher than the ideal level, which I understand is under 5.0, but as I've lost more weight since then (about 2st 9lb in total), it may well be that my cholesterol has gone down some more.

> 'My relationship with food has improved a lot and that I don't rely on it any more for comfort.'
> **Ana-Maria Hutchinson**

Finally, Club member Pam Prudence, who went through an early menopause and has to have a DEXA scan every five years, has seen an increase in her bone density after following the Amazing Inch Loss Plan. She wrote:

My bone density has improved by 1%, which is good, and it's down to the way I have changed my eating habits and the amount of exercise I do at your classes.

4 Are you ready to diet?

You have bought this book, so I have to assume you are serious about wanting to lose weight and get fitter. But how committed are you? What has prompted your decision to shed some pounds or kilos? Self-awareness is really important and you need to identify the triggers that can trip you up and the motivators that will keep you focused on the job in hand once you embark on the diet.

Rushing into the diet without planning your campaign may not give you the results you want. Investing in a little time to assess your frame of mind and get yourself properly organised before you start could provide the key to your ultimate success.

If you find yourself saying to your friends 'I really **ought** to lose weight' or 'I **should** lose weight' and you only bought this book to show willing, you are probably being pushed into considering a weight loss plan by a third party rather than making your own decision to take action. But if you are saying '**I have decided I am going to lose weight**' and '**I am going to get fitter**' you are much more likely to succeed.

Changing the way you think about food is imperative. One of the dangers of embarking on a weight loss plan is that you can become obsessed with food. As soon as you have had one meal, you are already planning the next … and the next! Food can take on a very unhealthy importance in your mind, which almost certainly will lead to failure as you will convince yourself

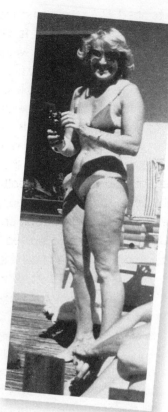

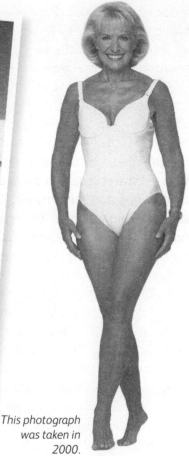

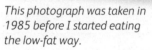

This photograph was taken in 1985 before I started eating the low-fat way.

This photograph was taken in 2000.

that you feel hungry and deprived – because you are thinking about food all the time! This needn't happen and you can retrain your brain, like I did.

Years ago when I was struggling with my own weight, I was obsessed by food – buying it, cooking it, tasting it, bingeing, dining out . . . In fact, food controlled my life. It was a nightmare. The more I tried to lose my unwanted weight, the more weight I gained. From originally only having a stone to lose, I ended up with almost 2½ stone to shed. Not a vast amount, I admit, but to someone who was only 5ft 2in tall it was significant. I hated the way I looked and my excess weight destroyed my self-esteem and affected every day of my life.

So what changed? In 1986, when I was forced on to a low-fat diet to avoid surgery for gall bladder removal, my eating habits were transformed. I had to avoid high-fat foods and found that when I cut out obvious fats like butter and cream from my diet, I lost loads of inches effortlessly. It was like a miracle. When I realised I could eat three decent-sized, healthy meals a day and keep my weight down and my body lean, I stopped seeing food as 'the enemy'. Instead, food took on a more positive role as a health-giving fuel that my body used as energy. My attitude to food changed completely and now food sits very happily in the back of my mind – rather than at the front. Consequently, I maintain my weight (within a pound or two) with very little effort.

I don't follow a 'diet' as such, but I eat low-fat foods as a matter of course. If my waistband becomes a little tight, I simply cut back for a couple of days and do a little more exercise and those extra inches quickly disappear. It works for me, so please let me help you get to this healthy point of balance too.

Most probably you will have to change the way you think about food, like I did, and you must be prepared to take action. You may need to change some behavioural patterns too. But if you have the will to do it, you can. It's all about **attitude**.

Take some time to ask yourself a few questions and have a notepad ready to jot down any thoughts or feelings. You don't have to show these to anyone else, but having them written down in black and white will help you to see more clearly how you think and feel and they will act as a useful reference point in the future. When you reach your goal weight, you'll be able to remind yourself how you felt when you started the diet and that could help you to stay slim in the long term.

Answer the following questions and jot down any thoughts and feelings:

Why do you eat the way you do?
What happened or changed in your life to cause you to gain weight?
Why do you want to lose weight?
How do you think you will feel when you have lost your excess weight?

You should find the chart on the facing page helpful as you prepare yourself for action. Why not copy it and open a folder or keep a notebook to record your progress notes? Establishing your determination to succeed is really important and you need to do everything possible to prevent lapses in your progress as you go along.

Next, it is really important to write down your goals – even those not associated with your weight or fitness. I do this all the time, as it keeps me focused and I achieve so much more that way.

Once you have reached this stage and thought about why and how badly you want to lose weight, you will have made a positive decision to do just that, as well as to get fitter and change your life for the better. You have accepted that you will have to make some changes (because if you don't you'll just get bigger) and that the likely rewards far outweigh the relatively small sacrifices you may have to make to achieve your goal.

When you have thought through your goals and the benefits you will be able to enjoy when you are slimmer, you'll find that sticking to a diet and fitness plan is relatively easy. The key is to accept responsibility and be accountable for your

Preparing to take action

List the positive aspects of following a healthy, low-fat diet and taking regular exercise (e.g. weight loss, less strain on joints, more energy, increase in confidence):

List the negative aspects of following a healthy, low-fat diet and taking regular exercise (e.g. will have to cut back on chocolate):

_____   _____
_____   _____
_____   _____
_____   _____
_____   _____
_____   _____

WHY do you want to change?
(Make a list, e.g. I want to be slim for my children; for my health; to be able to buy nice clothes)

_____   _____
_____   _____
_____   _____
_____   _____
_____   _____

HOW will losing weight make you feel?
(Make a list, e.g. more attractive, less tired, more confident, fitter)

_____   _____
_____   _____
_____   _____
_____   _____
_____   _____
_____   _____

decisions and, ideally, find support through a class or online group. It is definitely harder to lose weight on your own.

Every week, I hear stories from members of our Rosemary Conley Diet and Fitness Clubs and our online club about how losing weight has transformed their lives – not just in a small way, but dramatically. I feel so lucky to have played a small part in helping these people achieve their new, happier and more successful lives.

Losing weight increases our self-confidence. The more confident we are, the happier we become, and the happier we are, the more we get out of life in whatever form we choose to find it. In this book I want to build your confidence and make you feel like the woman (or man) you truly want to be. I want you to be happy in your own skin and to have a sunny outlook towards your future. We only have one life, so let's make the most of it!

Developing a positive attitude

Having a positive mental attitude is crucial to your success and you may find the following guide useful in helping you to develop a more positive attitude to your weight and fitness progress. The following acrostic was created by Caroline Whiting, Head of Training at Rosemary Conley Diet and Fitness Clubs, and she teaches it to our franchisees:

A Action required
T Take responsibility
T Turn fears into focus
I Imitate excellence
T Transform negatives into positives
U Uncover your hidden talents
D Develop yourself
E Expect the unexpected

Caroline then went a stage further and thought it would be interesting to work out where each letter of the word 'attitude' sat in the alphabet:

A = 1
T = 20
T = 20
I = 9
T = 20
U = 21
D = 4
E = 5

Add them all together and, amazingly, they come to 100! So, take these suggestions on board and enjoy 100 per cent success!

Before you start

Next, it's time to sort out your fridge and get rid of all those foods that are high in fat and that you really don't need if you're serious about losing weight. Pass them on to a slim and needy friend (or stick them in the freezer). Alternatively, just phase them out over the next week or two.

Take a look at the menu suggestions for each day of the 28-day programme and make a shopping list. The menus contain straightforward recipes and meal suggestions that require no special preparation. Your cuisine can be as simple or complicated as you choose.

5 How to lose a stone in a month

The 28-day programme in this book is designed to help you through the first four weeks of your weight and inch loss journey by offering you motivation, a daily diet plan and a progressive exercise programme which you can do with me each day by logging onto www.rosemaryconley.tv/ailpDay1. In addition to the daily toning exercises, I will also ask you to undertake some aerobic activity to ensure that you burn extra calories to maximise your rate of weight loss. By the end of the month, you will be significantly slimmer, stronger and fitter and you will be amazed at how different you feel.

For the first two weeks of the diet, the regime is quite strict in order for you to achieve a notable weight loss in this first fortnight. This will act as a tremendous motivator, as you will see a real change in how your clothes fit you, particularly around your waistband. The abdomen is a key target area for weight loss, because having a large waist size can pose a serious risk to your health.

In trials we have undertaken, the **average** weight loss of the trial dieters was 7.25lb after two weeks and an average of 14lb after four weeks. So I am confident that if you have a fair amount of weight to lose, you will lose a stone in the first month. If you have only a relatively small amount of weight to lose, then you will still see a significant drop in your weight and inches in the first 28 days.

There is absolutely no doubt in my mind that if you stick rigidly to the plan and undertake the exercises as recommended, you will be both surprised and thrilled at the results. The diet really does work and you will feel like a new person in just one month.

The diet is divided into three phases:

Phase 1: 14-Day Fast Track
Phase 2: 14-Day 1400
Phase 3: Your Personal Inch Loss Plan

The **14-Day Fast Track** diet is based on 1200 calories a day for the first two weeks. It is perfectly safe to eat this relatively low number of calories for a short, sharp kick-start of the diet. Next comes the **14-Day 1400** diet, which is slightly less strict and offers you an extra 200 calories a day – 100 to be used for a low-fat dessert or low-fat treat, plus 100 for an alcoholic drink, e.g. a 125ml glass of wine, or a high-fat treat, such as chocolate.

On Day 29, after the initial four-week diet and exercise plan, if you have more weight to lose, you can move on to the third phase: **Your Personal Inch Loss Plan**. By checking the charts on pages 378–9, you will be able to work out your personal calorie allowance based on your weight, gender and age. This allowance will be equivalent to your basal metabolic rate (BMR), which is the number of calories that you, as an individual, burn each day just to stay alive. If you continue to

---

If at any time you want to give your weight loss a boost after a period of overindulgence, for instance after a holiday or Christmas, you can return to the **14-Day Fast Track diet**. It is not to be followed long term unless your BMR determines that 1200 calories is the correct number for your daily needs, which might be the case if you are over 60 or have a small frame, or both.

diet on that number of calories, reducing the calories slightly as you lose each half stone, and you also take regular exercise, you will keep losing weight until you reach your goal.

The eating plan is based on low-fat, low-Gi foods (which keep you feeling fuller for longer), with some high-protein meal options (which have a high satiety value), and is combined with a daily exercise programme that will speed up your rate of weight loss, tone your muscles and boost your metabolism. There are plenty of delicious meal options for both meat-eaters and vegetarians. All the meals have been carefully selected to maximise volume and satisfaction while minimising calories and fat. Many of the recipes are ideal for entertaining and, I promise, your guests won't feel they are being presented with 'diet food'.

Why do we count calories?

Whether you follow a high-protein diet or a high-carb diet, calories do count. A 'calorie' is a term used to measure the energy value (fattening power) of food and drink. Different types of foods contain different amounts of calories, and foods that are high in fat contain the most. Depending on our age, gender and weight, the body uses about 1200–1400 calories a day just to fuel basic bodily functions (renewing and repairing body tissue, maintaining heart and lung function, and so on). Any physical activity you do throughout the day uses extra calories on top of this basic requirement. The more you move about, the more calories you will spend, and if you undertake formal physical exercise you will increase your calorie expenditure significantly, depending on the type of activity you do, how long you do it for and at what level.

On a weight-loss plan you need to consume sufficient calories to meet your everyday metabolic needs from healthy, nutrient-rich foods. This diet plan will give you all the nutrients

Reading nutrition labels

Check the nutrition labels on each food product before you buy. Look at the column that gives a 100-gram breakdown for the food, then check the figure for TOTAL fat content (see sample label). All foods containing five grams or less fat per 100 grams can be eaten as part of this Amazing Inch Loss Plan, providing you stay with your daily calorie allowance.

The fat content may be broken down into polyunsaturates and saturates, but on a weight-reducing diet, this is not significant. It is the total fat content per 100 grams that is relevant in your calculations. If you follow the simple five per cent fat rule, the fat content of your food will look after itself.

Remember, keeping an eye on the calories is just as important as checking the fat content. On the nutrition label look at the TOTAL CALORIES (KCAL) PER SERVING, alongside the ENERGY breakdown, to keep tabs on your daily intake.

NUTRITIONAL INFORMATION

typical values	amount per 100g	per 300g serving
Energy	443 kj/ 105 kcal	1329 kj/ 315 kcal
Protein	6.9g	20.7g
Carbohydrate (of which sugars)	11.2g (2.6g)	33.6g (7.8g)
FAT (of which saturates)	3.7g (1.7g)	11.1g (5.1g)

Even though there is a total of 11.1g fat in each serving, there is still only 3.7g fat per 100g (3.7%), making it a low-fat food.

As you can see, this food contains 315 calories per 300g serving. Keep this figure in mind when planning your menus.

you need and the exercise you do will help to maintain your metabolic rate as well as burn extra calories to help you lose weight faster and tone up. However, I would always recommend that you take a multivitamin supplement daily in case there is a nutrient or food group that you choose not to consume.

Each day, the average woman spends in total about 1800–2200 calories (for men the figure is between 2300 and 2700) in the maintenance of basic bodily functions and in going about her daily activities. The total calorie expenditure depends on your age, weight and activity levels. If you eat fewer calories than your body uses during the day, your body has to find the extra calories to fuel its needs from somewhere else – somewhere other than food – so it draws on its fat stores, which are situated around the body, to make up the difference and the result is you lose weight. Think of your body as a bank: if its current account runs out of funds, it has to draw some cash (calories) out of its savings account (fat stores) to make up the difference.

It is really important that you consume sufficient calories to meet your basic metabolic requirements (between 1200 and 1400 for the average woman) and if you do that by eating a diet that gives you enough calories to meet that basic need, it means that every bit of activity you do – and that includes normal day-to-day moving about as well as formal exercise – will be spending fat out of your body's 'savings account' of fat and you will become slimmer. And the more exercise you do, the more fat you spend! That's why diet and exercise is so effective.

Why low fat?

Gram for gram, or ounce for ounce, fat contains twice as many calories as carbohydrate or protein, so if you eat lots of high-fat foods, you will be taking in lots of calories. Quite simply, we become fat because we eat too much fat.

Interestingly, the fat we eat is stored on our bodies to be used as an 'emergency' energy (calorie) reserve so that in times of famine we can survive for longer. Carbohydrate and protein foods are easily used by the body for fuel, but fat is 'put into storage' and is only utilised as fuel once the calories from carbohydrate and protein have been exhausted.

If you reduce the amount of fat you eat, you will be putting less fat into storage and you will get leaner. And it doesn't matter whether it is saturated or unsaturated fat – both types have the same number of calories and will be stored around your body in the same way.

When you are trying to lose weight, I recommend you aim to eat foods that have no more than five per cent fat content (that's five grams of fat per 100 grams of food), with the exception of oily fish such as salmon or mackerel once or twice a week as these contain important nutrients for heart health. If you don't eat oily fish, take a fish oil supplement instead. Some lean meats may be slightly higher than five per cent too, as are raw oats.

On my low-fat diets, I estimate the average fat intake is somewhere between 20 and 40 grams per day, whereas in the average Western diet the figure is over 100 grams. Remember, my diets are low-fat, not fat-free.

Why low Gi?
Gi stands for 'glycaemic index'. The glycaemic index was originally created to help diabetics select the most effective foods to maintain their blood glucose levels. Some foods give a sudden sugar 'rush', which causes the body's blood sugar levels to rise rapidly and then drop quickly later, and this can be dangerous for diabetics. These foods are given a 'high' Gi rating.

Other foods release energy more slowly, giving a gentle and longer-lasting rise in glucose levels and then a very gradual fall, which is ideal for diabetics. These slow-energy-releasing foods have a 'low' Gi ranking.

In addition, doctors found evidence of improved heart health in diabetics who followed a low-Gi diet. So it was established that eating a low-Gi diet was good for everyone, not just diabetics. Soon there was a deluge of books published on the subject and low-Gi eating became very fashionable. Nevertheless, it is accepted by nutritionists and doctors alike that eating a diet rich in low-Gi carbohydrates is good for all of us.

LOW-GI CHOICES

- **Bread** Choose brown wholegrain or multigrain bread or bread made from stoneground flour. Pitta bread is also low Gi.
- **Pasta** All pasta is low Gi. Eat it with low-fat, tomato-based sauces in preference to creamy ones when you are trying to lose weight.
- **Rice** Basmati rice is the best choice as it has a lower Gi than most other types.
- **Potatoes** Choose sweet potatoes in preference to old ones. Waxy new potatoes are also low Gi. Cook and eat them with their skins intact to add fibre to your diet.
- **Breakfast cereals** Go for high-fibre cereals (like All-Bran, Bran Buds, Grape Nuts and Fruit 'n' Fibre) or cereals containing wholegrain (e.g. Shredded Wheat and Special K). Oat-based varieties (such as porridge or muesli) are usually low Gi. Watch out for 'cluster' types of cereal as these can contain a lot of extra fat and sugar.

For the dieter, eating a diet rich in low-Gi foods is very helpful, as the very nature of low-Gi foods is that they help keep blood sugar levels stable and keep you feeling fuller for longer, which is ideal for anyone on a reduced-calorie eating programme. And eating low Gi is easier than you think. Just make some simple low-Gi choices when shopping for carbohydrates and include these in your menus, and you will automatically be eating a low-Gi diet.

Why exercise?

Exercise burns extra calories, which helps us to lose weight faster. **Aerobic** exercise – that's any exercise which makes us breathe more deeply and take in extra oxygen – burns fat from our body's fat stores as fuel, so it should always be included in a weight-loss programme. Moreover, aerobic exercise increases our metabolic rate, not just during the activity itself but also for several hours afterwards. Each day on this programme I ask you to do some aerobic activity and once a week I ask you to do a 45–60 minute session, which could be an aerobics class or working out to a fitness DVD at home.

Toning and **strength** exercises make our muscles stronger and give us a better shape. As muscle tissue is energy-hungry, the stronger our muscles, the higher our metabolic rate and the more efficient our bodies will become at burning fat. On six days a week in this plan I ask you to do a few specific exercises that target the major muscles in the body. The toning sessions only take about five minutes and they become more challenging throughout the 28 days. These workouts can be found on www.rosemaryconley.tv/ailpDay1 for each day of the plan. If you follow the programme closely you will be amazed at how quickly you progress to the more difficult exercises that will prove even more effective at toning your muscles and giving you a great figure. They really will transform your body!

There is a real synergy between aerobic and strength exercise. During aerobic exercise, the extra oxygen that we breathe in through our lungs is transported around the body and into our muscles via the bloodstream. Muscles contain thousands of little engines called 'mitochondria' which 'fire up' during aerobic exercise, but to do this they need fuel. So the mitochondria 'power houses' call on the fat stores around the body and, with the help of the extra oxygen from the aerobic activity, they burn that fat for fuel. The result is the fat burns in the oxygen flame, and we use up some of our stored body fat!

The stronger our muscles, the more mitochondria we grow and the more fat we can burn. That's why combining aerobics with toning and strength exercises is so effective in helping us achieve a leaner body and it also helps to keep our bones healthy and strong.

For some years we have been encouraged to work out aerobically five times a week for around 30 minutes. But not everyone has the time to go for a 30-minute walk on five days a week and it really doesn't have to be as time-consuming as it first appears.

The reason why we are encouraged by the experts to work out aerobically (such as going for a brisk walk) for 30 minutes is because it increases our heart rate, which is good for our overall fitness and health. However, the good news is that we don't have to do 30 minutes to see benefits; if we work at a higher intensity, we can increase our heart fitness in a much shorter period of time. For instance, running for 10 minutes or dancing for 15 minutes has an equivalent benefit to our health and burns around the same number of calories, but most importantly is 'do-able' within our busy lifestyles.

We are all familiar with the importance of having our five portions of fruit and/or vegetables a day, and the five-a-day slogan has become universally understood and recognised.

Now I am keen to promote the notion of doing our 'five-a-week' exercise. I'd like to encourage people to become more conscious of adding up the physical activities they undertake over the period of a week – activities which would constitute the equivalent of five 30-minute sessions, but in real time could be completed in significantly fewer minutes if done at a higher intensity.

On page 351–2 I have listed a variety of sports and activities that deliver a similar benefit to our health and fitness as a 30-minute walk. Check out the list and see which activities you might enjoy doing and then think of ways to incorporate them into your weekly lifestyle. Do this and, before long, you will have developed a new habit of undertaking your 'five a week' and dramatically improved your health as well as significantly increasing your chances of living longer and more healthily.

In addition to our aerobic exercise, we should do some strength exercise on most days each week and this need only take as little as five minutes. If you do the exercises in this book, you will change your body from being a 'fat storer' into a 'fat burner' in no time and this will help you to stay slim in the long term.

The bottom line is that exercise makes us slimmer, fitter and healthier and gives us a better figure. Just do it!

All the classes at a Rosemary Conley Diet and Fitness Club include a 45-minute workout, which incorporates a combination of aerobic and toning exercises. For details of your nearest class visit www.rosemaryconley.com

What about alcohol?

Most people love having a drink with their friends and, indeed, some alcohol in moderation can be good for our health. I am the first to admit I love a glass of wine, so I am not about to tell you that you should give it up. 'Phew!' I hear you say. But problems arise when alcohol is drunk in excess and, for some people, it is the main cause of their weight problem.

Let's look at some facts. Alcohol contains a lot of calories that offer no nutrients. As alcohol is a toxin, the body will always process it quickly, burning it away as energy as a top priority before it processes the carbohydrate, protein and, of course, the fat that you've eaten. The consequence of this is that your half bottle of wine will have used up 250 calories of your daily allowance, and the excess calories from any food you have eaten will have been deposited as fat around your body rather than being burned away, because the calories from alcohol have jumped the queue and taken precedence.

The other factor is that alcohol weakens our willpower, so we are much more likely to say to ourselves, 'Oh, forget the diet today, I'll be good tomorrow!' Then to cap it all, when we drink a lot of alcohol we tend to fancy fatty foods! Crisps and peanuts, pizzas and curries are usual choices, with disastrous consequences for the dieter. If this is only a rare occurrence, that's fine, but if it happens regularly, you need to change your lifestyle if you are serious about losing weight!

Let's get started!

Step 1

Before you start this diet and fitness programme, make sure you have the appropriate food in the house and that you have discarded or donated any foods that might tempt you from the amazing benefits you are going to enjoy. Check that you have some suitable footwear for exercise and that you have told your family and friends what you are aiming to do. Enlist their support and encouragement. Tell them why you are doing this and that everyone will benefit if you lose your excess weight (you'll be much happier, which has to be of benefit to them!).

Step 2

Decide on your start day and weigh yourself first thing that morning and then again each week, at the same time of day and on the same scales. Measure yourself too, either using a tape measure or, if you have one, my Magic Measure®. This is a special tape measure that comes with a series of colour-coded, clip-on tags, some permanent and some removable, and each colour represents a different part of the body (bust, waist, hips, etc.). You clip a permanent tag on to the tape measure to register your 'start' measurements, then at your future measuring sessions you clip a removable tag in the hole at your nearest inch measurement. This will enable you to see your progress from the first day of your weight and inch loss campaign.

If you don't have a Magic Measure®, take your measurements anyway on Day 1 and write them down on a piece of paper and, when you get your Magic Measure®, you can clip your 'start' markers on your 'start' measurements on the tape accordingly. Alternatively, just make a note of your details at the back of this book or in your notebook or folder.

Step 3

Before you start the programme, take a photograph of yourself (or ask someone else to take it) wearing something unflattering. This photo is going to inspire you to stick with the programme and also give you incredible encouragement as you see your progress over the coming weeks and months. Take a new shot every four weeks and place them in your personal diet folder or notebook. You will be so glad you did when you reach your goal weight and you look back and see how far you've come. You never know, you might be selected to feature in my *Diet & Fitness* magazine – and some of you might even make it to the front cover! To be considered, you will have to write to me with full details of your weight and inch loss and any relevant stories, enclosing clear 'before' and 'after' shots and your contact information.

All the slimmers who are featured in the magazine come to our head offices at Quorn House, in Leicestershire. We go shopping to choose the clothes for the day, then return to the studio at Quorn House where each slimmer has a makeover with a professional make-up artist before being photographed by one of the UK's top photographers. To finish off the day, I interview them for Rosemaryconley.tv, our television channel on the web. It is a magical day and everyone really enjoys themselves.

We are always inspired when we meet these successful slimmers and hear their amazing stories – and next year, it could be you!

How to follow the 28-day programme

During the first two weeks of the **14-Day Fast Track** diet, you are allowed three meals a day – one breakfast, lunch and dinner – plus two power snacks, one mid-morning and one mid-afternoon. You can follow the diet menus I have suggested, or choose any breakfast, lunch or dinner in this book. In addition you should consume 450ml (¾ pint) skimmed or semi-skimmed milk, which you can take on cereals and in teas and coffees as you wish throughout the day. I ask you not to drink any alcohol during these first two weeks. Sorry – but it is only for this short period (you'll be able to enjoy a drink in week three) and going without for these two weeks will have a dramatic effect on your weight loss.

From week three, on the **14-Day 1400** diet, you can have an extra 200 calories a day (1400 in total). So, in addition to your three meals and two power snacks, you can enjoy an alcoholic drink or a high-fat treat like chocolate or crisps (max. 100 kcal) plus a low-fat pudding or treat (max. 100 kcal). If you wish, you can save up your 'treat' calories over a week (max. seven days, 700 calories) for a bigger, high-fat treat or a night out on the town! Of course, you may also choose to use these 'treat' calories for low-fat food. It's up to you.

All the meal suggestions are calorie-counted and all are interchangeable within each category, providing you swap like for like, e.g. one breakfast for another breakfast, and aim to include five portions of fruit and/or vegetables each day. The diet plan I recommend is a balanced one, but because our personal needs vary, I recommend that you take a multivitamin supplement daily to ensure you get all the vitamins you need. If you have a set of my Portion Pots® (these are handy tools for measuring everyday foods such as breakfast cereals, rice and pasta quickly and accurately), use them to measure your portion sizes – don't guess or you may overestimate your serving sizes and end up not losing as much weight as you expect to. For readers who don't have a set I have given the equivalent metric measures.

Cook without fat and don't add any fat during your food preparation. Grill or dry-fry foods instead of frying (or use a little spray oil). When cooking vegetables, rice and pasta, add a vegetable stock cube to the cooking water for extra flavour.

Follow the toning exercises by logging on to www.rosemaryconley.tv/ailpDay1 and do the aerobic challenge as suggested for the first 28 days. The toning programme is progressive, so each day the exercises become more challenging. As you proceed through the programme, if you find it difficult to complete the more advanced moves, just repeat the earlier versions of the exercises until you feel ready to progress.

Diet notes

Milk
Make sure you consume 450ml (¾ pint) skimmed or semi-skimmed milk a day for use on breakfast cereals and in teas and coffees. If you are allergic to or intolerant of cow's milk you may have soya or rice milk instead. If you don't drink much milk, you may substitute 125ml low-fat yogurt (max. 75 kcal) for 150ml (¼ pint) milk.

Bread
Choose wholegrain, multigrain or stoneground bread. In these menu plans, one slice of wholegrain bread has 100 calories.

Breakfast cereals
Choose high-fibre cereals (e.g. All-Bran, Fruit 'n' Fibre, Bran Buds and Grape Nuts) or ones containing wholegrain (such as Shredded Wheat and Special K). Oat-based varieties (e.g. porridge or muesli) are usually low Gi. Watch out for 'cluster' types of cereal as these can contain a lot of extra fat and sugar.

Fruit and vegetables
Aim to eat five portions of fruit and/or vegetables each day. A portion of fruit is one small orange, apple or pear or a regular kiwi fruit, nectarine or peach or 115g fruit such as berries or grapes. In the diet plan this is described as '1 piece fresh fruit'. Approximately 1 × 115g serving of vegetables counts as one of your 5-a-day portions. All vegetables should be cooked and

served without added fat. 'Unlimited vegetables' means any vegetables except potatoes.

Salad
Salad includes all salad leaves, cress, tomatoes and raw vegetables such as cucumber, peppers, carrots, onion, mushrooms, celery and courgettes, and may be served with any low-calorie, fat-free dressing, balsamic vinegar or soy sauce. Avoid pre-packed or ready-made salads with dressing as most are high in fat.

Gravy
Make gravy with gravy powder or low-fat granules.

Oily fish
For good heart health it is important to eat two portions a week of oily fish, e.g. mackerel, salmon, sardines, herrings, even though this exceeds my five per cent fat ruling.

Drinks
Regular and fruit teas and coffee made with water are unrestricted. Use milk from your daily allowance as required. All low-calorie and diet drinks may be drunk freely. Water is also unrestricted – aim to drink about 2 litres a day.

 means suitable for vegetarians or vegetarian option is available.

 means suitable for freezing.

 means this is a high-protein meal choice.

Remember, all meals are interchangeable within each category, so you can swap or repeat your favourites as you wish.

Throughout this book, I occasionally mention products or services that help people to lose weight and get fitter. At Rosemary Conley, we spend a lot of time and effort to find gadgets, products and services that we genuinely believe will help you on your weight loss journey. Everything has been personally chosen by me, whether it be a pedometer, a set of Portion Pots®, my Magic Measure® or a milk jug, and nothing is offered unless I am satisfied that it is of a high standard. If at any time our goods or services do not meet those high standards, please let me know.

Rosemary Conley Mature Cheese is a superb product, which tastes just like full-fat Cheddar but with half the calories and just five per cent fat. It is only available to order or through our classes. Log on to www.rosemaryconley.com for details.

6 The 28-day plan

Weeks 1 and 2
Phase 1: 14-Day Fast Track

Weeks 3 and 4
Phase 2: 14-Day 1400

Daily allowance

Throughout the diet the calories have been allocated as follows:

Breakfast	200 kcal
Mid-morning Power Snack	50 kcal
Lunch	300 kcal
Mid-afternoon Power Snack	50 kcal
Dinner	400 kcal
450ml (¾ pint) skimmed or semi-skimmed milk	200 kcal
Total (Weeks 1 and 2)	**1200 kcal**

Add-ons from Week 3

1 alcoholic drink OR high-fat treat	100 kcal
1 low-fat dessert OR low-fat treat	100 kcal
Total (Weeks 3 and 4)	**1400 kcal**

Phase 1: 14-day fast track
Day 1

This is an exciting day! It marks the start of one of the most important journeys of your life. That might sound dramatic, but imagine how different you will look and feel in one month! As you continue on the programme you will realise that losing weight is life-changing, and you have already taken the first big step.

Have you read Chapter 5? If not, please do so now before you begin this programme. Otherwise it's like buying a new gadget and ignoring the instructions in your haste to get started. These pages contain vital information on how the programme works and how to maximise your progress.

I hope you enjoy today's menu. If there's a meal suggestion you don't fancy, feel free to flick through the book and find an alternative meal in the same category (e.g. swap a lunch for another lunch option) to suit your taste and your lifestyle. That's the beauty of this diet, it's so versatile.

Find a suitable time to do the exercises to fit them around your other activities. If you are really busy, it's a good idea to do them first thing, before you shower, so they don't get squeezed out of your schedule later. Exercising first thing will also strengthen your willpower throughout the rest of the day. Just log on to www.rosemaryconley.tv/ailpDay1. Today's five-minute tone-up targets the waist, abdominals, backside, chest and those horrible flabby underarms! Make sure you warm up first. Alternatively, if you plan to do the exercises later in the day, you could do them after walking the dog or vacuuming your living room, as activities like this will also warm up your body.

Have you weighed and measured yourself? If not, do it now. Lastly, find an old belt and, using a marker pen, make a mark on the belt where it fits around your waist and write today's date on it too. Or consider ordering a Magic Measure® (www.rosemaryconley.com). If you join one of our classes, you'll receive one free in your membership pack.

MENU

Breakfast
■ 2 well-grilled back bacon rashers or 2 Quorn sausages, grilled, served with 1 dry-fried medium-sized egg, 3 tomatoes, halved and grilled, and 5 grilled mushrooms ☑ Ⓟ

Mid-morning power snack
■ 150g strawberries ☑

Lunch
■ 1 × 400g can any soup (max. 150 kcal and 5% fat). Plus 1 Müllerlight yogurt, any flavour (max. 150 kcal)

Mid-afternoon power snack
■ 1 rice cake spread with 20g Philadelphia Extra Light soft cheese and sliced cucumber ☑

Dinner

■ Pasta Bolognese: Dry-fry 100g lean minced beef or Quorn mince in a non-stick pan, seasoning well with black pepper. Drain off the fat, add ½ chopped onion, 1 crushed garlic clove and ½ chopped red pepper and dry-fry until soft. Stir in ¼ jar Dolmio Bolognese Original Light Pasta Sauce and 1 × 200g can chopped tomatoes and simmer for 10 minutes. Serve with 1 yellow Portion Pot® (45g uncooked weight) pasta shapes, boiled with a vegetable stock cube ☑
OR
■ Black Bean Prawns (see recipe, p.255) served with 1 blue Portion Pot® (55g uncooked weight) or 1 red Portion Pot® (144g cooked weight) boiled basmati rice. Plus 1 Marks & Spencer meringue nest topped with 1 tsp 0% fat Greek yogurt and 1 tbsp raspberries

FIVE-MINUTE TONE-UP

See www.rosemaryconley.tv/ailpDay1

AEROBIC CHALLENGE

Go for a 20-minute walk and then do the stretches on p.343 to finish or go to www.rosemaryconley.tv/stretches.

Exercise tip

Make sure you wear comfortable fitness gear and always wear trainers during aerobic exercise to protect your feet, legs and joints. Always warm up before you start and then stretch at the end of your workout.

MOTIVATIONAL THOUGHT FOR THE DAY

Take a really good look at yourself in the mirror today, wearing just your underwear, so that you can face up to your body and where you are now, then confirm to yourself that this is the first day of a journey towards a new you. Say out loud that you are embarking on this weight loss plan for YOUR benefit, and no one else's.

Now I would like you to detach yourself from your reflection in the mirror and, instead of seeing yourself, think of that image as your new best friend, the one you are going to help to lose weight. Don't shy away from talking to that image in the mirror as you lose your excess weight and inches. Be encouraging and be complimentary. Look at the good features of this new friend – maybe their eyes, skin, hair, face, nails, or even their feet. It is important to get rid of any feelings of self-loathing you may have and to start respecting this person, who is totally worthy of your friendship and support. It's much easier to have respect for yourself if you see yourself as another person. From now on, stop being negative or putting yourself down – you wouldn't do that to a friend – and start complimenting yourself. Become your own best friend.

Day 2

I hope that yesterday went well and that you managed to stick to the diet and do the exercises. You probably slept better than usual as you won't have felt so bloated or lethargic and the extra exercise should have helped too. Avoid popping on the scales just yet – wait until next week when the difference will be more noticeable and you will get a more accurate result. Our weight can fluctuate from one day to another, so weekly weigh-ins are more helpful than daily ones.

If you are not normally a breakfast-eater, hopefully you managed to eat at least something before 10 a.m. People who eat breakfast tend to weigh less than those who don't, so please make the effort to get into the habit.

You will need a sturdy dining chair for today's toning exercises, which will work the waist, backside, thighs and the posture muscles. Although these exercises take only five minutes, they are really effective. To do the exercises with me, log on to www.rosemaryconley.tv/ailpDay2.

* Rosemary Conley mature cheese contains 5% fat and is available by mail order via www.rosemaryconley.com

MENU

Breakfast
- 1 green Portion Pot® (50g) Special K cereal plus milk from allowance and 1 tsp sugar ✓

Mid-morning power snack
- 12 seedless grapes ✓

Lunch
- 100g cooked chicken breast (no skin), sliced, served with a large mixed salad and 1 tbsp Hellmann's Extra Light Mayonnaise **P**

OR

- 1 × 50g wholemeal pitta bread filled with 50g low-fat houmous and chopped mixed salad sprinkled with low-fat dressing of your choice ✓

Mid-afternoon power snack
- 20g low-fat cheese* (max. 5% fat) plus 5 cherry tomatoes ✓

Dinner
- 1 × 115g (raw weight) salmon steak, steamed or microwaved, served with 80g boiled new potatoes (with skins), plus 1 yellow Portion Pot® (70g) frozen or canned peas, 100g steamed broccoli or asparagus and 1 tbsp Hellmann's Extra Light Mayonnaise

OR

- 1 low-fat veggie burger (max. 180 kcal and 5% fat, e.g. Grassington's Vegetable Quarter Pounder or Quorn Quarter Pounder) cooked as per instructions. Serve with 115g boiled new potatoes (with skins) and a large salad tossed in low-fat dressing ✓

FIVE-MINUTE TONE-UP

See www.rosemaryconley.tv/ailpDay2

AEROBIC CHALLENGE

Walk up and down stairs 3 times consecutively. Do this 4 times in total throughout the day.

Exercise tip
Every bit of physical activity you do burns extra calories, so make an effort to move about more in your everyday life. Use the stairs more, park your car further away from the office or shops, take a walk at lunchtime, offer to carry bags and boxes for colleagues – it all adds up and will help you to lose weight faster.

MOTIVATIONAL THOUGHT FOR THE DAY

It can be really motivating to read how other people have succeeded in losing weight and turning their lives around. You'll find real-life slimming success stories in my *Diet & Fitness* magazine or you can watch the slimmers being interviewed on www.rosemaryconley.tv. One day these people resolved to do something about their weight, just like you. They decided enough was enough and that they were going to make some changes – and they did. Four of our 2011 Slimmers of the Year are featured in this book. They followed this diet to the letter, and the weight fell off them.

One of the most important factors that determines who is featured in my magazine is the quality of a slimmer's 'before' photograph. I know we hate having our photograph taken if we are overweight – I didn't even have one of myself when I was at my biggest – but it will demonstrate how far you have come once you have reached your goal weight. It is that dramatic transformation that inspires other potential dieters to take action. So, if you have not taken your before photograph yet, please do so today.

Have you found yourself a notebook or folder for recording your notes and observations of how you feel? It's really good therapy as you progress on your weight loss journey as it will act as a constant reminder of your achievements.

Day 3

Every day is important but today is really important. It's the day your body starts drawing on its 'savings account' of fat to make up the deficit left by the reduction in your daily calories and the increase in your physical activity.

During the first couple of days of a diet, it's likely that your body is still processing some of the food you ate before you started the diet, alongside the restricted calories from this 14-Day Fast Track diet, and you will also be burning some of the carbohydrate stored in your liver and muscles. But from today, your body will only be using the calories from the food you are now eating to fuel essential bodily functions, and the resulting shortfall in calories needed for the extra activity you are doing is being drawn from your fat stores. So, from now on, you will genuinely be getting slimmer.

Eating your between-meals power snacks will help you get through the morning and afternoon without hunger pangs, but if you find you are not hungry at any of these times, save these calories for when you do feel like a nibble. For instance, I have my breakfast at 6.30 a.m. and I am always really hungry by lunchtime at 12.30 p.m., but then I can easily go right through to my next main meal at 7 p.m. without feeling hungry. However, I like to have a little something, usually a tiny portion of cereal, before I go to bed at 10 p.m. We are all different, so make the diet work for you.

Log on to www.rosemaryconley.tv/ailpDay3 for today's toning exercises which will work on the abdominals, back, inner thighs, underarms and chest, and the aerobic activity will burn fat.

MENU

Breakfast
- 1 Müllerlight yogurt, any flavour (max. 150 kcal), plus 1 small banana

Mid-morning power snack
- 1 × 200g slice melon (weighed without skin) ☑

Lunch
- 1 pitta bread, split open, then spread with low-fat Marie Rose dressing or very low-fat mayonnaise and filled with shredded lettuce, cherry tomatoes and 100g cooked prawns
OR
- 1 × 300 pack Rosemary Conley Solo Slim® Tomato Soup (order from www.rosemaryconley.com), plus 1 slice wholegrain bread ☑

Mid-afternoon power snack
- 1 Rakusen's cracker topped with 1 × 20g triangle Laughing Cow Extra Light soft cheese, plus 5 cherry tomatoes

Dinner
- Quick and Easy Chicken Curry: Dry-fry 1 × 115g chopped chicken breast (no skin) or Quorn chicken-style fillets in a preheated non-stick pan with ½ chopped onion and 1 crushed garlic clove. Sprinkle 1 tsp curry powder over and 'cook out' for 1 minute, then add 1 small chopped chilli, ½ chopped green pepper, 25g button mushrooms (optional) and 1 × 400g can chopped tomatoes, and simmer for 5 minutes to reduce. Serve with 1 blue Portion Pot® (55g uncooked weight) or 1 red Portion Pot® (144g cooked weight) basmati rice ☑

OR

■ 3-egg omelette made using milk from allowance and cooked in a non-stick pan. Add 25g grated Rosemary Conley low-fat Mature Cheese and 25g shredded ham or chicken. Serve with a large salad tossed in fat-free dressing **P**

FIVE-MINUTE TONE-UP

See www.rosemaryconley.tv/ailpDay3

AEROBIC CHALLENGE

Work out at an aerobics class or to a fitness DVD for 30 minutes or go for a 30-minute walk.

Exercise tip

When doing strength exercises, always work your muscles to the point where they feel tired, then do five more reps. This way, you challenge the muscle fibres and they become stronger. It is these extra reps that do the real work.

MOTIVATIONAL THOUGHT FOR THE DAY

Writing down our goals and ambitions is really important if we are serious about achieving them, and it's the same when trying to lose weight and get fitter.

Back in the 1950s, the Board of Governors at Yale University in the US decided to survey all their final-year students to establish their lifestyles, eating habits, religious beliefs, hobbies, and so on. One of the questions asked was 'Do you have any goals?'. As this was one of the top universities in the US, the Board was somewhat surprised to learn that only 10 per cent of students admitted to having goals. Next, the questionnaire asked if the students had written down those goals. Only four per cent said they had.

Twenty years later, the university thought it would be interesting to find out how the original group of students had progressed since they completed the study. It took a year to track them all down and one or two had died, but all those still living completed the new survey. The most interesting factor to emerge was that the four per cent who had said they had goals and had written them down, were *each* earning more than the *total* earnings of the remaining 96 per cent!

So, determine your goals and write them down. It works! You can always revise your goals, add to them, and remove any that become unimportant, but having a goal to aim for keeps you focused and helps to keep you on track.

Day 4

You should be feeling slimmer today. When you woke up this morning did your stomach feel a little flatter? And when you got dressed, hopefully your waistband felt less tight and your clothes looser. It's a great feeling!

The temptation at this point is to think that you have the diet sussed and that you don't need to measure the quantities of food you eat, but trust me, you do. Portion control will make a big difference to your overall rate of weight and inch loss. If you don't already own a set of my Portion Pots®, check them out on www.rosemaryconley.com. They are unique, inexpensive and incredibly effective. And if you join one of our classes or our online club, you will receive a set free in your membership pack.

Today's toning exercises focus on the waist, stomach, backside and outer thighs and your posture muscles in the upper back. Log on to www.rosemaryconley.tv/ailpDay4 for today's workout. Be as active as you can and stick strictly to the diet plan. If you do, the rewards will be fantastic.

MENU

Breakfast
- 1 yellow Portion Pot® (125ml) fresh orange juice, plus
1 slice wholegrain bread spread with 2 tsps marmalade, jam
or honey ☑

Mid-morning power snack
- 2 dried apricots ☑

Lunch
- 2 low-fat beef or pork sausages (max. 5% fat) or 2 Quorn
sausages, grilled, served with 1 yellow Portion Pot® (115g)
baked beans, 1 dry-fried small egg, 1 small can tomatoes
boiled well to reduce, plus unlimited grilled or boiled
mushrooms ☑ P
OR
- Chicken Noodle Soup (see recipe, p.242) served with 1 small
wholegrain pitta bread, toasted

Mid-afternoon power snack
- 1 kiwi fruit plus 5 seedless grapes ☑

Dinner
- Chinese Chicken Kebabs (see recipe, p.243) served with 1
blue Portion Pot® (55g uncooked weight) or 1 red Portion Pot®
(144g cooked weight) basmati rice per person
OR
- 1 low-fat pizza (max. 350 kcal and 5% fat, e.g. Marks &
Spencer Count On Us) served with a mixed salad tossed in
fat-free dressing ☑

FIVE-MINUTE TONE-UP

See www.rosemaryconley.tv/ailpDay4

AEROBIC CHALLENGE

Go for a cycle ride for 20 minutes or cycle on a stationary exercise bike for 10 minutes, plus either walk briskly for 30 minutes at some point in the day or go for a 20-minute swim.

Exercise tip

If you watch television in the evening, why not use the time during the ad breaks or the breaks between programmes to walk up and down stairs three times. Do this four times in an evening and it will burn a significant number of calories and tone your bottom too!

MOTIVATIONAL THOUGHT FOR THE DAY

Research has shown that keeping a written record of what we eat and drink can affect how much weight we lose. In trials, slimmers who wrote down what they ate and drank, lost twice as much weight as those who didn't.

The reason why keeping a written record is so helpful is because it makes us accountable. We can very conveniently forget what we've eaten and swear blind that we have been saintly with our dieting regime, convincing ourselves that we really have! Writing down what you eat, as you eat it, is a great habit to get into and it will help you to understand your temptations and identify the times when you are most vulnerable to straying from the diet. It's for this reason that I have created a 'Handbook' to accompany this diet in which you write down everything you eat and drink, and the exercise you do, so you can then look back and see why you did so well one week and not on another. It's well worth the investment of effort.

Day 5

Well done for getting this far on the 14-Day Fast Track. If you are still sticking strictly to the diet and the exercises, you stand an extremely high chance of long-term success. If you were going to fail, you would have fallen by the wayside yesterday.

Three or four days into a diet is when slimmers are likely to feel peckish on occasions and not make time for the exercises. They may also be missing some of their favourite fattening foods or alcohol. However, if you want to regain your youthful figure and feel years younger in the next month or two, it's going to take determination, dedication and discipline. It's not difficult, though, if you have the right attitude and the will to succeed. The rewards for staying focused and disciplined are huge and I want you to picture yourself succeeding and looking fabulous in that new outfit you are going to wear when you reach your goal.

Today I'm giving you a rest from the toning exercises, but I would like you to do some extra aerobic exercise to boost your fat burning and weight loss. Look at my suggestions and select an activity you enjoy and don't forget to drink plenty of water before, during and after exercising.

Remember, nothing tastes as good as being slim feels!

MENU

Breakfast
■ 1 slice wholegrain bread, toasted, topped with 1 yellow Portion Pot® (115g) baked beans ☑

Mid-morning power snack
■ 1 blue Portion Pot® (14g) Special K cereal (eaten dry or with milk from allowance) ☑

Lunch
■ Large salad of grated carrots, beansprouts, chopped peppers, celery, tomatoes, cucumber and red onion, served with 130g canned tuna chunks (in brine) or 1 blue Portion Pot® (100g) low-fat cottage cheese, plus 1 tbsp Hellmann's Extra Light Mayonnaise. Plus 1 low-fat yogurt (max. 100 kcal and 5% fat) ☑ P

Mid-afternoon power snack
■ 100g cherries

Dinner
■ Chilli Prawn Stir-Fry with Peppers and Mushrooms: Dry-fry 150g fresh prawns in a non-stick wok. When they have changed colour, add ½ each chopped red and green pepper, 5 button mushrooms, 1 chopped celery stick, ½ chopped red onion, 1 small courgette, chopped, and ½ pack of fresh (or 1 whole can) beansprouts. Do not overcook. Just before serving add 1 tbsp Thai sweet chilli dipping sauce and soy sauce to taste P
Plus 1 low-fat yogurt or other low-fat dessert (max. 100 kcal and 5% fat)

OR
- Ham, Leek and Sweet Potato Pie (see recipe, p.253) with unlimited vegetables (excluding potatoes) or salad
OR
- Leek and Sage Meatballs with Pasta (see recipe, p.258) ☑

FIVE-MINUTE TONE-UP

Rest day.

AEROBIC CHALLENGE

Exercise aerobically for a minimum of 30 minutes today. Select one of the following or create a combination of activities that you can do one after the other for 30 minutes in total:

- Swimming
- Brisk walking
- Cycling
- Aerobics (class or DVD)
- Heavy housework (vacuuming, cleaning windows, bed making, etc.)
- Cardio equipment in the gym (e.g. stepper, cross trainer, bike, treadmill)

Warm up first and then, after your chosen activity, cool down by just gently walking on the spot for 2 minutes, then stretch out at the end of your workout (see pp.343–7) to avoid aching muscles tomorrow.

> **Exercise tip**
> When you go for a walk, include a few jogging steps every hundred yards, then walk again for another hundred yards. Turn your walk into a walk/jog and you will burn significantly more calories and see a dramatic improvement in your fitness.

MOTIVATIONAL THOUGHT FOR THE DAY

We all need encouragement when aiming for a goal and never more so than when we are trying to lose weight. It may be that your husband or partner is a real 'encourager', but if they aren't, you need to find someone who is!

If you go to one of our diet and fitness classes you will be surrounded by encouragers and that could be a good place to find a diet buddy. For members of our online club, the online chatroom and coffee shop offer the perfect opportunity for encouraging each other. Alternatively, you might find someone at work who is interested in your progress and will help to support and encourage you when the going gets tough, or maybe you have a mum or sister who will be brilliant at the job. It doesn't matter who it is, as long as you have someone who is positive and interested in you.

When you do find your encourager, explain to them how much you value their interest and encouragement. We all like to feel needed but we don't like to overstep the mark, so it's important to let the encourager know how much they are appreciated and that they are doing a useful job.

Day 6

After today, there's only one more day to go before the first week's weigh-in. Now is the time to be extra vigilant at avoiding temptation and to work especially hard at the exercises. I have increased the intensity of the exercises today so that you burn extra calories and fat. This is now the big push to maximum weight and inch loss at the beginning of Day 8.

Don't be tempted to skip meals as you will only end up feeling so hungry you'll be tempted to grab anything to eat! So eat your meals and your Power Snacks and do your exercises. Today's five-minute tone-up will work on your waist, back, inner and front thighs and your chest. Log on to www.rosemaryconley.tv/ailpDay6. If you stick to the diet and do the exercises, I PROMISE you will lose weight. Have a good day.

MENU

Breakfast

▪ 1 yellow Portion Pot® (30g) fruit and fibre cereal served with milk from allowance and topped with 1 red Portion Pot® (115g) fresh raspberries or 1 tsp sugar ☑

Mid-morning power snack

▪ 1 Ryvita spread thinly with Philadelphia Extra Light soft cheese ☑

Lunch

▪ 1 pre-packed sandwich of your choice (max. 300 kcal and 5% fat) ☑
OR
▪ Broccoli and Leek Soup (see recipe, p.240) served with a small granary roll ☑

Mid-afternoon power snack

▪ 10 cherry tomatoes, plus chunks of carrots, cucumber and pepper ☑

Dinner

▪ Spicy Chicken Pasta: Dry-fry 110g chopped chicken breast (no skin) and ½ chopped onion in a non-stick wok and season with freshly ground black pepper. Add 1 crushed garlic clove, 1 sliced green pepper, 1 × 400g can chopped tomatoes, ½ small chopped chilli and a dash of Worcestershire sauce and allow to simmer for 5 minutes. Serve with 1 yellow Portion Pot® (45g uncooked weight) or 1 red Portion Pot® (110g cooked weight) pasta shapes
OR

■ Sweet and Sour Quorn: Dry-fry ½ × 350g pack Quorn Chicken Style Pieces (175g) with ½ chopped onion, ½ each chopped red and green pepper, 5 button mushrooms, halved, 1 chopped celery stick and 1 small chopped courgette ☑️🅿️ Plus 1 low-fat yogurt or other dessert (max. 100 kcal and 5% fat)

FIVE-MINUTE TONE-UP

See www.rosemaryconley.tv/ailpDay6

AEROBIC CHALLENGE

Take a brisk walk for 30 minutes at some point during the day.

Exercise tip
When doing toning or strength exercises, always breathe out on the 'effort', e.g. when lifting your head and shoulders on an abdominal curl, and breathe in as you return to the start position. And remember to keep breathing! Holding your breath for more than just a few seconds when exerting yourself can be dangerous.

MOTIVATIONAL THOUGHT FOR THE DAY

Be watchful of the temptation to sabotage your dieting efforts and find an excuse for breaking your diet and fitness programme. This is a common trait in people who are frightened of failing. If you have tried to lose weight before but didn't get the results you'd hoped for, you might be tempted to overeat or drink too much alcohol just before weighing day so you can say, 'Well I would have lost much more, but I had to go to Caroline's birthday celebration and that's why I've not lost as much as I should have.' Deliberately – though often subconsciously – ruining your chances of success is very destructive.

The diet will work if you stick to it and the exercises will tone you up and burn fat if you do them so that you lose fat and inches. Please trust the diet and don't even consider sabotaging your progress. Stay focused and think about how you will feel at the end of the programme if you stick to it, and the scales will reward you. The bonus is that you will gain confidence, which will help you as you progress towards your goal. You really have nothing to lose but your weight and inches, so go for it!

Day 7

Well done for reaching this stage. With your weighing and measuring day coming up tomorrow you need to put every bit of effort into the exercises in order to maximise your success on the scales first thing in the morning.

Today's diet offers lots of bulk as I don't want you feeling hungry and being tempted off track. Your body is now in full fat-burning mode, so every bit of willpower you can summon will pay dividends. Should you get hungry and be tempted to stray, remember that your body is drawing calories out of its savings account of fat.

Before my evening meal I always have two large glasses of diet ginger beer. I love it and it curbs my appetite so that I'm not overly hungry when I sit down to eat my main meal of the day. It works for me. If you are really hungry by the time you start eating, you'll find the amount of time it takes you to eat your meal isn't long enough for the food to reach your stomach and register that you've had enough. So try to eat slowly and drink plenty of water or low-calorie drinks to allow time for your brain to receive that 'I'm full' signal.

Today's toning exercises are more challenging and are designed to work the muscles in your waist, abdomen, backside, outer thighs and underarms. Log on to www.rosemaryconley.tv/ailpDay7 for your workout. Your muscles are becoming stronger every day, so feel the muscles 'working' as you do each exercise.

MENU

Breakfast
- 2 Quorn sausages, grilled, served with 1 medium-sized dry-fried egg and 1 × 200g can tomatoes, boiled until reduced ✔ P

Mid-morning power snack
- 20g sultanas ✔

Lunch
- 200g 2% fat Greek yogurt mixed with 1 tsp runny honey and 1 red Portion Pot® (115g) raspberries or chopped strawberries or 1 yellow Portion Pot® (70g) blueberries, topped with 1 tsp muesli ✔ P
OR
- Greek Salad Wrap (see recipe, p.266) ✔

Mid-afternoon power snack
- 100g fresh pineapple ✔

Dinner
- 150g roast chicken breast (no skin) served with 100g dry-roast sweet potatoes plus 200g other vegetables of your choice (e.g. carrots, broccoli, cauliflower) and low-fat gravy
OR
- 2 Quorn Lamb Style Grills, grilled, served with 115g boiled new potatoes (with skins), plus 200g other vegetables of your choice and a little low-fat gravy and mint sauce ✔

FIVE-MINUTE TONE-UP

See www.rosemaryconley.tv/ailpDay7

AEROBIC CHALLENGE

Go for a brisk 30-minute walk or work out to a fitness DVD, such as my Real Results DVD, for 30 minutes. Also, walk up and down stairs 4 times consecutively, twice during the day. Really go for it today!

Exercise tip

It's important to have some water close by when exercising. Taking regular top-ups of water during aerobic exercise has been proven to be very effective in helping us to keep going for longer, for instance when exercising on a treadmill or exercise bike.

MOTIVATIONAL THOUGHT FOR THE DAY

Having reached this stage, you have taken a very big step towards a new you. Starting a diet and fitness campaign properly prepared, and then completing the first week, is a major achievement. The delight you will feel tomorrow when you step on the scales will give you an enormous boost and this will set you up for the next seven days. After you have completed the 14-Day Fast Track your calorie allowance will be increased according to your age, gender and weight, but sticking to the 1200-calorie allowance during this first phase of the diet will give you a fantastic start in your weight loss campaign. Research has shown that if we make significant progress early in our dieting campaign, we are far more likely to continue on the diet because we have already witnessed the inches disappearing and our clothes are feeling looser.

Make a real effort with the exercises today. I have given you some additional aerobic fat-burning activities to help you burn extra calories and fat and maximise the results for tomorrow. If you want to do even more, that's great. Stick to the diet, watch your portion sizes and don't cheat! You'll be so glad tomorrow.

Day 8

By the time you read this you will already have weighed and measured yourself. Make sure you write down your results. Try on your measuring belt and mark on it your new waist measurement. If you have a Magic Measure®, clip on your second set of tags and see how much you are shrinking. Add up the total number of inches (or centimetres) you have lost and look at the equivalent measurement on a ruler. It is fascinating to see the inches end to end in a straight line!

Hopefully, you will have lost a significant amount of weight too. Now find yourself a carrier bag and place in it some tins of food or packets of dried food of the equivalent weight that you have lost this week. Keep them in that bag and stash it away in a cupboard or under the stairs to be brought out this time next week or any time in between when you need a motivational boost and a reminder of what you have achieved so far.

Just one more week to go on this very strict diet. Stick with it and you will be the winner! Today's toning exercises will work your abdominals a little harder than before. I have also included an exercise that works your backside and your inner thighs at the same time and another that works your chest and underarms simultaneously, plus one for your shoulders and one for your back. Don't rush them but do them carefully to make them more effective. I've given you a break from your aerobic exercise today, so enjoy the rest!

Remember, all meals in each category are interchangeable.

MENU

Breakfast

▧ Tomatoes and Mushrooms on Toast: Boil 1 × 400g can chopped tomatoes well to reduce to a thick consistency and season well with freshly ground black pepper. Spoon onto 1 large slice toasted wholegrain bread and serve with 10 grilled mushrooms ✔

Mid-morning power snack

▧ 1 red Portion Pot® (115g) raspberries topped with 2 tsps low-fat yogurt ✔

Lunch

▧ 2 hard-boiled eggs served with salad of chopped vegetables and salad leaves, tossed in low-fat dressing of your choice. Plus 1 kiwi fruit and 1 small pear ✔ P
OR
▧ Turkey and Mango Samosas (see recipe, p.247) served with unlimited fresh vegetables or salad

Mid-afternoon power snack

▧ 150g fresh fruit salad ✔

Dinner

▧ Beef Kebabs: Cut 150g rump steak into bite-sized pieces and thread on to wooden skewers with 8 chestnut mushrooms, then baste with 50g tomato passata and 1 tsp balti curry paste. Cook the kebabs for 5–6 minutes in a health grill or 10 minutes under a conventional grill. Check the centre of meat is cooked and, when ready to serve, sprinkle with ½ tbsp chopped fresh coriander and serve with fresh green vegetables or salad P

OR
■ Any low-fat ready meal (max. 400 kcal and 5% fat, including accompaniments) ☑

FIVE-MINUTE TONE-UP

See www.rosemaryconley.tv/ailpDay8

AEROBIC CHALLENGE

Rest day.

Exercise tip
It is really important to warm up before exercising as this helps to increase circulation and prevent injury and muscle soreness later. Although it's tempting to get going with any fat-burning exercises straight away, you will burn fat more efficiently if you have warmed up your muscles first. Remember, we burn fat in our muscles, so it makes sense to get your muscles (with their little engines called mitochondria) firing on all cylinders by the time you come to the fat-burning exercises in the aerobic section.

MOTIVATIONAL THOUGHT FOR THE DAY

Here are five tips to keep you on track this week.

1   Use your Portion Pots® or weigh out your daily portions of cereal, rice and pasta, etc., to ensure you stay within your calorie limit.

2   Remove the skin and fat from any poultry or meat before you put it on your plate, or before cooking if appropriate.

3   Avoid spreading butter, margarine or spread on your bread, as this adds loads of unnecessary calories. Instead, use low-fat sauces such as tomato ketchup, HP Fruity Sauce or very low-fat mayonnaise.

4   Dry-fry foods in a non-stick frying pan or wok. You can prepare many delicious low-fat dishes this way (e.g. stir-fries, curries, soups), and add any liquid or cooking sauces later, depending on the recipe.

5   Have a long drink before you start eating to help fill you up. Only cook the amount of food you need and serve it on a slightly smaller dinner plate than usual so that it looks like a generous serving size. This avoids waste and the temptation to go for second helpings.

Day 9

Now that you're into the swing of things for week two of the 14-Day Fast Track you are probably feeling quite excited. You are already past the halfway stage of this really strict couple of weeks and your body is getting used to eating healthier – and less – food than before. You are sleeping better, you wake up more rested and are feeling fitter. You have to be, as you are eating healthy foods, exercising regularly, your muscles are working harder and the aerobic exercise will have made your heart and lungs more efficient. Well done and keep up the good work!

Today's toning exercises, which are done with the help of a chair, will work your waist, stomach, outer and front thighs and your shoulders. Log on to www.rosemaryconley.tv/ailpDay9 for your workout.

MENU

Breakfast

- 1 Weetabix or Shredded Wheat served with milk from allowance plus 1 tsp sugar and 1 thinly sliced medium banana ✔

Mid-morning power snack

- 1 medium pear ✔

Lunch

- 1 Batchelors Cup a Soup. Plus 1 Müllerlight yogurt (max. 150 kcal) and 1 kiwi fruit

OR

- 1 × 175g oven-baked sweet potato topped with 75g baked beans, served with a side salad tossed in fat-free dressing of your choice ✔

Mid-afternoon power snack

- 1 blue Portion Pot® (75g) tomato salsa served with 1 carrot, 1 celery stick and 1 × 5cm piece cucumber, all sliced into crudités ✔

Dinner

- Cheesy Quorn Bake: Dry-fry 1 finely chopped red onion and 1 crushed garlic clove in a non-stick pan until soft, then stir in 100g Quorn mince and cook for a further 2 minutes. Add 200g chopped tomatoes, 250g tomato passata, ½–1 tsp vegetable stock powder, ½ tbsp chives and reduce to a gentle simmer. While the Quorn mixture is simmering, heat a non-stick griddle pan and cook 150g chopped courgettes on both sides until lightly browned, seasoning with black pepper. Layer the

courgettes and Quorn mixture in an ovenproof dish. Pour 150g 2% fat Greek yogurt over the top and add 25g grated Rosemary Conley low-fat Mature Cheese (or vegetarian alternative) and black pepper to taste. Bake in a preheated oven at 200C, 400F, Gas Mark 6 for 20 minutes until the cheese has melted and the dish is hot all the way through. Garnish with chopped chives ☑ 𝐏
OR

■ Lamb and Mushroom Goulash (see recipe, p.251) served with green vegetables

FIVE-MINUTE TONE-UP

See www.rosemaryconley.tv/ailpDay9

AEROBIC CHALLENGE

Go for a brisk walk or swim or a bike ride for 30 minutes.

Exercise tip
Yesterday I talked about the importance of warming up before exercise. Today, I want to emphasise the vital role of cooling down and stretching after your workout. During a workout, you are challenging your muscles and this can produce a build up of lactic acid and cause your muscles to ache later – sometimes two days later. Stretching the muscles you've used in your workout will help to eliminate this discomfort.

MOTIVATIONAL THOUGHT FOR THE DAY

Does your stomach feel flatter this morning and your clothes looser? Soon you will need to buy some new clothes. I did hear of one slimmer 'hanging on' for as long as possible before buying a smaller size only to have their trousers fall down one day as they walked down the street!

Rather than investing in new clothes that are only going to fit you for a short while, why not have a look in a charity shop or dress agency for something nice to wear temporarily. I always take my clothes to one of these outlets when I'm bored with them or I've had second thoughts after buying them and felt that, after all, they didn't do a lot for me. Sometimes brand new, or at least nearly-new clothes, can be found in charity shops and there are real bargains to be had. And when you drop down to the next dress size, you can take the first lot back and buy some new, smaller ones. I suggest you only invest in new clothes when you reach your ultimate goal.

One important thing, though. Make sure you keep at least one – your largest – garment as a reminder of how big you once were, as you will forget later when you get used to being slim.

Day 10

Ten days into the 14-Day Fast Track diet and you may be feeling peckish. I have tried to select low-Gi foods to keep your blood glucose levels stable and help you feel fuller for longer. Be sure to eat your power snacks and drink plenty of fluids. Often hunger can be confused with dehydration, so keep well hydrated.

When I trialled this low-Gi diet I was surprised at how well the women and men who followed it coped with the very restricted calorie allowance in the first two weeks. They all said they hardly felt hungry during that time and were amazed at how much healthier they felt in such a short time. The feelings of general wellbeing they reported were significant. So stick with the diet and do the exercises every day and soon you will feel like a new person too.

Today is an aerobic day so there are no toning exercises. Do make sure you find time to do your fat-burning aerobics, though, to help speed up your weight loss.

MENU

Breakfast
■ ½ fresh grapefruit plus 1 medium-sized poached egg served on 1 small slice toasted wholegrain bread spread with Marmite ☑

Mid-morning power snack
■ 1 yellow Portion Pot® (125ml) apple juice ☑

Lunch
■ 100g cooked chicken breast (no skin), sliced, and served with a large mixed salad and 1 tbsp Hellmann's Extra Light Mayonnaise **P**
OR
■ Stir-Fried Rice Noodles (see recipe, p.264) served with salad ☑

Mid-afternoon power snack
■ 75g sliced mango ☑

Dinner
■ 1 × 150g (raw weight) lean pork steak (all fat removed), grilled, served with 115g boiled new potatoes (with skins), 200g other vegetables of your choice, plus low-fat gravy and 1 tbsp apple sauce
OR
■ 1 × 300g pack Rosemary Conley Solo Slim Spicy Vegetable and Lentil Dahl (order from www.rosemaryconley.com). Served with a small salad. Plus 1 low-fat yogurt (max. 120 kcal and 5% fat) ☑

FIVE-MINUTE TONE-UP

Rest day.

AEROBIC CHALLENGE

Do 40 minutes of aerobic work, choosing one of the following activities: working out to a fitness DVD or at an aerobics class, swimming, cycling, brisk walking or using cardio equipment at the gym (e.g. stepper, treadmill, cross-trainer, exercise bike).

> **Exercise tip**
> When we do aerobic exercise, the fat-burning takes place in our muscles. The stronger our muscles, the more fat we burn, so it's important to make the effort to keep our muscles strong. Using a toning band or light handweights is a great way to increase the intensity of a toning workout.

MOTIVATIONAL THOUGHT FOR THE DAY

When we lose weight and burn body fat it's important to look after our skin so that it 'shrinks' with us and doesn't end up being saggy. There will be some natural shrinkage and then, when we exercise, the extra blood pumping around the body close to the skin's surface warms the skin, making it more metabolically active and more toned. It works like magic in helping our skin to firm up.

When I meet slimmers who have lost massive amounts of weight – 10 stone is not uncommon – I always ask about their skincare routine. They tell me that they moisturise and massage their skin every morning after showering and this, combined with all the exercise they did to achieve their amazing weight loss, had a remarkable effect on their skin.

In 2008 I decided to ask a manufacturer if they could develop an inexpensive body toning and moisturising body cream that would be effective at helping skin to shrink back on a weight loss plan. I told them I wouldn't put my name to it unless it was proven to work. A cream was developed, put through a clinical trial and launched later that year. It has proved extremely popular with readers and members of our clubs alike, even in minimising stretch marks, and the feedback has been very positive (see www.rosemaryconley.com).

But, remember, any body lotion massaged into your skin is better than none and will have some effect in helping your skin to contract and stay healthy.

Day 11

I hope your encourager is supporting you and that you are sharing your thoughts and feelings with them. And how are you getting on talking to yourself as a third party? Are you saying positive and encouraging things to yourself and affirming your progress to date? You didn't become overweight overnight and you won't get slim overnight either, so be patient and think forward, upward and onward.

Remember, you can choose meals from anywhere in this book as long as you substitute a lunch for a lunch or a dinner for a dinner. It doesn't matter which one you select. The important thing is that you enjoy what you are eating.

In today's exercise programme I've focused on the abdominals, backside, inner and front thighs, and the chest and underarms, so log on to www.rosemaryconley.tv/ailpDay11 for today's workout. Practise these exercises regularly and you will see a significant difference in your muscle strength and your overall body shape.

MENU

Breakfast
- 2 large bananas ☑

Mid-morning power snack
- 1 yellow Portion Pot® (125ml) fresh orange juice ☑

Lunch
- Spread 2 slices wholegrain bread with HP Fruity Sauce (or similar) and make into a sandwich with 3 grilled turkey rashers, then toast in a sandwich toaster or double-sided electric grill
OR
- Garlic Mushroom Pasta (see recipe, p.260) ☑

Mid-afternoon power snack
- 2 satsumas ☑

Dinner
- Spicy Pork Steak: Mix together 1 tsp ground cumin, 1 tsp ground ginger and 1 tsp smoked paprika on a plate, then press 300g lean pork steak into the spices and season with salt and pepper. Cook the steak in a health grill for 8–10 minutes or under a conventional grill for 8–10 minutes each side. Serve hot with a mixed salad or vegetables of your choice 🄿
OR
- Vegetable Chilli: Dry-fry 1 chopped onion in a preheated non-stick pan. Add 1 × 200g can mixed beans in chilli sauce and 1 × 200g can chopped tomatoes plus chopped vegetables (e.g. courgettes, mushrooms, carrots, peppers) and simmer for 15–20 minutes. Serve with 1 blue Portion Pot® (55g uncooked weight) or 1 red Portion Pot® (144g cooked weight) basmati rice ☑

FIVE-MINUTE TONE-UP

See www.rosemaryconley.tv/ailpDay11

AEROBIC CHALLENGE

Walk up and down stairs 4 times consecutively and repeat 4 times during the day.

Exercise tip

If you want a flat stomach, you need to do plenty of toning exercises such as stomach crunches and ab curls in order to strengthen your abdominals. However, these exercises in themselves will not get rid of the fat, but when you do your aerobic exercise, your stronger abdominal muscles will encourage fat burning from around the whole body much more efficiently and that includes the abdominal area.

MOTIVATIONAL THOUGHT FOR THE DAY

I am a firm believer in only weighing and measuring ourselves once a week however tempting it might be to pop on the scales midweek. The problem is that fluctuating body fluid levels and all manner of other factors can affect our weight. If you were to weigh yourself now, you might find you've made great progress but then see little difference between now and your weigh-in session on Day 15, and you will only be disheartened. So please be patient and wait until the 'official' weigh-in day – and then you can celebrate!

Scales should be placed on a flat, non-carpeted surface for greatest accuracy, but keep them out of the bathroom. Bathrooms are damp and steamy and this can affect the mechanism in the scales. Body fat monitors are very popular now and are an easy way to see how much body fat you have lost. However, only check your body fat reading monthly or, better still, bi-monthly as, again, the reading can vary, depending on your body's fluid levels, and an occasional reading is likely to be more significant and encouraging. Do not use a body fat monitor if you are pregnant or have a pacemaker fitted, as body fat monitors work by passing a tiny electric current through the body. Fat acts as an electrical insulator, while muscle conducts the current very efficiently. The voltage drop across the body therefore depends on the relative amounts of fat and muscle.

Measuring the different areas of your body with a tape measure is important too, because when we are exercising regularly we sometimes lose inches without losing weight. All that matters is that we are getting smaller.

Day 12

Only three days to go before the end of this 14-Day Fast Track! The feeling of satisfaction and achievement when you reach Day 15 will be amazing. From then on, you will have the opportunity to enjoy treats, alcohol and puddings! But for now, you must concentrate on this last run on the homeward straight. Stay focused, exercise loads, drink plenty of water or low-cal drinks and DON'T CHEAT!

Today's toning exercises focus on the waist and stomach area, the inner and outer thighs, and the shoulders. Log on to www.rosemaryconley.tv/ailpDay12 to work out with me.

MENU

Breakfast

▪ 1 Quorn bacon-style rasher, grilled, served with 1 yellow
Portion Pot® (115g) baked beans plus 1 tomato, halved and
grilled, and 50g grilled mushrooms ☑ℙ

Mid-morning power snack

▪ 2 kiwi fruit ☑

Lunch

▪ Prawn Wrap: Spread 1 tortilla wrap with 1 tsp Thai sweet
chilli dipping sauce, then fill with 50g cooked prawns, chopped
salad leaves, peppers, cucumber, celery and cherry tomatoes
and wrap into a parcel before cutting in half horizontally to
make 2 wraps
OR
▪ Large salad of grated carrots, beansprouts, chopped
peppers, celery, tomatoes, cucumber and red onion, served
with 1 blue Portion Pot® (100g) low-fat cottage cheese, plus
1 tbsp Hellmann's Extra Light Mayonnaise; followed by
1 low-fat yogurt (max. 100 kcal and 5% fat) ☑

Mid-afternoon power snack

▪ 1 small bowl of mixed salad tossed in fat-free dressing ☑

Dinner

▪ Lamb Stir-Fry: Cut 150g lean lamb steak into strips and
dry-fry with ½ chopped onion and ½ crushed garlic clove in a
non-stick pan over a high heat for 1–2 minutes. Add 1 tsp mint
sauce, 75g stir-fry vegetables and ½ tbsp soy sauce and toss
well before cooking for 7–8 minutes. Serve on a bed of lightly
cooked beansprouts ℙ

OR
■ 2 Quorn sausages, grilled, served with ½ pack readymade cauliflower cheese (max. 200 kcal and 5 % fat) and green vegetables of your choice ☑

FIVE-MINUTE TONE-UP

See www.rosemaryconley.tv/ailpDay12

AEROBIC CHALLENGE

Go for a brisk 30-minute walk and aim to clock up at least 10,000 steps on your pedometer. Alternatively, walk up and down stairs 5 times consecutively and repeat later in the day.

Exercise tip
One of the most effective ways to trim inches from your waist is to use a hula hoop or do a Salsacise workout. Moving the hips from side to side in a fast but small and controlled movement works the waist and abdominal muscles. I had never had such a small waist as when I was training for my first Salsacise DVD.

MOTIVATIONAL THOUGHT FOR THE DAY

Today would be a good day to flick through some fashion magazines or catalogues and think about what type of clothes you'd like to wear when you are slim. Slipping on a dress that is several sizes smaller than you used to wear will give you so much pleasure.

Would you consider yourself to be an 'apple' shape (large tummy and slim arms and legs), a 'heart' shape (large busted with slim legs and arms) or a 'pear' shape (small bust, narrow waist and large hips, thighs and arms)? It is helpful to recognise what type of shape you are and then dress accordingly. By making careful clothes choices you can address any imbalances you see in your figure, accentuating your good points and minimising the not so good ones.

Colours are really important too. Have you noticed that if someone tells you that a certain dress or top suits you, often it's the colour that has caught their eye. Learn which colours make you come alive and which ones don't. With a 'new you' in the making, it is worth using every ace in the pack to make sure you look your absolute best.

Day 13

For the next two days I am going to encourage you to step up your aerobic activity quite significantly. In addition to doing today's toning exercises, which focus on the waist, back, outer and front thighs and shoulders, I would like you to take every opportunity you can to be active. Walk up and down stairs whenever you have time, or go for an extra-brisk walk or jog. Be ultra-good with your food portion sizes and don't 'guesstimate'.

Try to stay busy so you don't get bored and start thinking about food! Avoid going food shopping for the next couple of days if you can – you might be tempted to buy something you'll regret.

MENU

Breakfast
▓ 2 eggs scrambled with milk from allowance and served with 100g grilled tomatoes and unlimited grilled mushrooms ☑Ⓟ

Mid-morning power snack
▓ 1 yellow Portion Pot® (70g) blueberries, topped with 1 tsp low-fat natural yogurt ☑

Lunch
▓ Homemade Vegetable Soup (makes enough for approx. 6 servings): Bring 2 litres of water to the boil in a large pan, then add 2 vegetable stock cubes and 400g peeled and trimmed vegetables (e.g. carrots, parsnips, onion, cabbage) or leftover vegetables and boil until cooked. Remove from the heat, add some chopped coriander and black pepper and leave to cool a little. Pour the soup in small batches into a food processor and blend for a few seconds, then transfer to a storage container or jug and allow to cool before storing or freezing. Reheat as required, allowing 300ml per serving and accompany with a slice of toasted wholegrain bread ☑

Mid-afternoon power snack
▓ 1 fat-free yogurt (max. 50 kcal) ☑

Dinner
▓ Oven-Baked Salmon: Place 1 × 110g salmon steak in an ovenproof dish, top with 1 tsp Thai sweet chilli dipping sauce and the juice of ½ lime. Bake in a preheated oven at 200C, 400F, Gas Mark 6 for 8–10 minutes, or until cooked. Serve with 100g boiled new potatoes (with skins) and unlimited green vegetables

OR

■ Prawn (or Quorn) Saag (see recipe, p.256) served with 1 green Portion Pot (170g) cooked egg noodles or 1 blue Portion Pot® (55g uncooked weight) or 1 red Portion Pot® (144g cooked weight) basmati rice per person ✔

Plus 1 meringue nest topped with 2 tbsps 0% fat Greek yogurt and 2 sliced strawberries

FIVE-MINUTE TONE-UP

See www.rosemaryconley.tv/ailpDay13

AEROBIC CHALLENGE

Work out for 30–40 minutes at an aerobics class or to one of my aerobic fitness DVDs (my latest Real Results Workout DVD is a great fat burner). Alternatively, go for a 40-minute brisk walk.

Exercise tip

Wearing wrist and ankle weights makes our arm and leg muscles work harder during toning exercises, but we should not use them during aerobic exercise as they can place too much strain on the joints, particularly the shoulders, or cause us to trip.

MOTIVATIONAL THOUGHT FOR THE DAY

Did you know that one pound of body fat is equivalent to half a litre of oil? So when you get weighed tomorrow, really appreciate every single extra pound that you have lost this week.

The great news is that, even after you have finished the 14-Day Fast Track, you will continue to lose weight at a very healthy and encouraging rate of two or three pounds per week while enjoying a more generous calorie allowance in weeks three and four.

Your body should be feeling comfortable with the amount of calories it is receiving – it won't feel it is starving and your metabolic rate should be staying buoyant, particularly in view of the amount of exercise you are doing. Remember, aerobic exercise raises the metabolic rate and it stays elevated for several hours afterwards, while toning exercises encourage stronger, energy-hungry muscles, which also results in a higher metabolic rate, so it's a win/win situation all round.

Day 14

Only one day to go to the end of the 14-Day Fast Track and your second weigh-in. Tomorrow's results will probably not be as significant as last week's because in the first seven days of dieting some of the weight you lost will have been fluid. By week two your fluid levels will have evened out, so what you are losing now is real, unadulterated body fat. However, the tape measure will tell you how many inches you have lost – and hence give you an indication of how much body fat has disappeared – and this should give you lots of encouragement.

Today, stay focused and avoid snacking at all costs. Work hard at your aerobic exercise and aim to complete all the reps in today's toning exercises, which work the abdominals, backside, front thighs, chest and upper arms and shoulders.

Try not to go food shopping until after you have weighed and measured yourself tomorrow, so you are not led into temptation. Have a great day.

Remember, if you find preparing your own meals too time-consuming, have a look at my Amazing Inch Loss Plan Solo Slim diet in chapter 12. We will deliver real meals that are already calorie counted to your door. Just add some veg or salad.

MENU

Breakfast

▓ Fruit Smoothie: blend 150g fresh fruit (peaches, strawberries, raspberries or blueberries) with 100g Total 2% fat Greek Yoghurt and milk from allowance ☑

Mid-morning power snack

▓ 1 kid's fun-size mini banana ☑

Lunch

▓ 1 × 175g oven-baked sweet potato, topped with 75g baked beans and served with a side salad tossed in low-fat dressing of your choice ☑

Mid-afternoon power snack

▓ 1 small apple ☑

Dinner

▓ Mixed Grill: 4 turkey rashers and 1 low-fat sausage, grilled, served with 1 dry-fried egg, 1 yellow Portion Pot® (115g) baked beans, unlimited grilled mushrooms plus 1 × 400g can tomatoes boiled well to reduce **P**
OR
▓ 3-egg omelette made using milk from allowance and cooked in a non-stick pan. Add 25g grated Rosemary Conley low-fat Mature Cheese and 25g shredded ham or chicken. Serve with a large salad tossed in fat-free dressing **P**

FIVE-MINUTE TONE-UP

See www.rosemaryconley.tv/ailpDay14

AEROBIC CHALLENGE

Take a 30–40-minute brisk walk or work out to a fitness DVD for 30–40 minutes. Don't forget to stretch afterwards.

Exercise tip

Did you know that we burn twice as many calories standing up than we do sitting down? So try to stand up when you are making phone calls or chatting.

MOTIVATIONAL THOUGHT FOR THE DAY

Today is a very important day. If you have managed to get to the end of this tough fortnight, with its restricted-calorie diet, and you've refrained from drinking alcohol and eating chocolate and completed the exercises every day, you are a star! Well done. You have achieved a significant goal and this will have boosted your self-esteem and confidence. Brilliant!

First thing tomorrow morning, after you have visited the bathroom, weigh and measure yourself carefully, then write down all the details in your notebook. Take a good look at yourself in the mirror and congratulate yourself on your progress. Even if you still have some way to go, you have done very, very well to get this far.

Remember not to sabotage your progress now. Keep focused and stay active for this last day of the 14-Day Fast Track.

Phase 2: 14-day 1400
Day 15

I hope you are delighted with the results that the scales and the tape measure or Magic Measure® have given you today. Move the portable clips on your Magic Measure® to today's measurements and add your inch losses to your total-inches-lost chart. Remember to try on your measuring belt too. Find your 'this-is-how-much-weight-I've-lost' carrier bag and add to it the appropriate weight of tins or packets of food equal to this week's weight loss. Be proud of your achievements and don't forget to tell your encourager.

From today you will be following the **14-Day 1400** diet and you are allowed an extra 200 calories each day. So you can have a low-fat pudding or some extra fruit up to the value of 100 calories, plus an alcoholic drink or a high-fat treat such as a fun-size Twix as long as it has no more than 100 calories.

The eating plan I've suggested for today includes a pudding and a treat of a glass (125ml) of champagne, because you deserve it. I suggest you buy a small bottle of champagne to avoid wastage – and temptation! – or why not invite some friends round to share a larger bottle and toast your success so far? Of course you can swap the champagne for another treat or drink if you want.

The exercises are getting much more challenging now to help you achieve the maximum benefit in this first month of your new diet and fitness regime. Today we'll be targeting the waist, back, inner and outer thighs and the chest and underarms. Do what you can and if you find any of them too tough, do the easier versions that you are already familiar with and then progress to the harder variations later. I have given you a rest day from your aerobics today.

MENU

Breakfast
- 200g Total 2% fat Greek Yoghurt mixed with 1 tsp runny honey ☑

Mid-morning power snack
- 1 whole papaya, peeled and deseeded ☑

Lunch
- Salad Bowl with Prawns, Chicken or Ham: Place a large selection of shredded salad leaves and fresh herbs such as coriander and basil in a serving dish. Add layers of chopped peppers, onion, celery, mushrooms, cucumber and cherry tomatoes and top with chopped fresh fruits such as pineapple, papaya, mango, kiwi. Add 50g cooked prawns or chicken or shredded ham, then pour some low-fat Marie Rose sauce or other low-fat dressing over the salad and sprinkle with chopped chives P
OR
- Any pre-packed sandwich (max. 300 kcal and 5% fat) ☑

Mid-afternoon power snack
- 100g cherries ☑

Dinner

■ 150g cod fillet, microwaved or steamed, and 50g cooked prawns, served with ½ × 300g pack (150g) Schwartz for Fish low-fat Chunky Tomato, Olive and Rosemary Sauce, plus unlimited carrots and broccoli or courgettes and 1 yellow Portion Pot® (70g) peas **P**
OR
■ Southern Fried Turkey (see recipe, p.246) served hot with unlimited vegetables (excluding potatoes) or salad **P**

Dessert

■ 1 × 165g Müllerlight vanilla yogurt sprinkled with dark chocolate

Alcohol or high-fat treat

■ 1 yellow Portion Pot® (125ml) champagne or white wine
OR
■ 1 × 25g bag Walkers Baked Salt & Vinegar crisps ☑

FIVE-MINUTE TONE-UP

See www.rosemaryconley.tv/ailpDay15

AEROBIC CHALLENGE

Rest day.

Exercise tip

By parking your car further away at the supermarket you are more likely to find a space and avoid getting your car scratched or dented. You will have walked extra steps towards your fitness and slimness too!

MOTIVATIONAL THOUGHT FOR THE DAY

'Nothing succeeds like success', so the proverb goes, and now that your weight and inch loss progress has taken a huge leap forward you should settle comfortably into the second phase of this weight loss programme.

While the next two weeks will be slightly easier because you have an extra couple of hundred calories each day to play with, in order to maximise your weight and inch loss, I want you to pep up your activity levels. In any case, you will be feeling fitter by now, as well as lighter, so you should be able to do more without feeling exhausted.

Put every bit of effort into this next 14 days and in two weeks' time you will have achieved a massive turnaround in your health and fitness. Enjoy it.

Day 16

I hope you enjoyed your alcoholic drink or high-fat treat yesterday and that it had a positive effect of making you feel good rather than frustrated that you couldn't have more! Some people find it easier to abstain completely rather than dice with temptation – once they have the taste of the alcohol or chocolate they find it difficult to stop – while others find that having a little of what they fancy is enough to keep them satisfied. I fall into the second category. I am quite happy to have a few chips from my husband Mike's plate, or just a spoonful of someone else's delicious dessert (Mike doesn't do desserts!). Fortunately I have an understanding husband and accommodating friends! So, recognise which sort of personality you are and plan accordingly. Avoid temptation and play to your strengths.

Try to do today's aerobic challenge with extra vigour so you burn even more calories and fat. Today's toning workout uses a dining chair and concentrates on the abdominals and hips and thighs. Log on to www.rosemaryconley.tv/ailpDay16 to work out with me. Your muscles are working much harder now, which will really help to tone your body. Remember to drink plenty of water or low-cal drinks to stay hydrated.

MENU

Breakfast
▧ 2 Quorn sausages, grilled, served with 1 × 400g can tomatoes boiled until reduced, plus 50g grilled mushrooms ✓ **P**

Mid-morning power snack
▧ 1 × 90g pack Tesco Fresh Apple and Grape Snack Pack ✓

Lunch
▧ Mixed Bean Salad: Mix together 100g drained, canned chickpeas, 100g red kidney beans and 25g sweetcorn kernels. Add 2 sliced spring onions, 3 halved cherry tomatoes, unlimited chopped celery, peppers and cucumber, and mix well. Stir in some chopped fresh coriander and basil and toss in balsamic vinegar or fat-free dressing of your choice and add freshly ground black pepper to taste ✓
OR
▧ 1 pack Rosemary Conley Solo Slim® Soup: choose from any flavour, including Lentil, Mushroom or Minestrone (order from www.rosemaryconley.com). Plus 1 slice wholegrain bread and 1 piece fresh fruit ✓

Mid-afternoon power snack
▧ 1 rice cake spread with 20g Philadelphia Extra Light soft cheese and sliced cucumber ✓

Dinner
▧ ½ pack any branded fresh filled pasta (max. 5% fat) served with ½ pot readymade low-fat fresh tomato-based sauce (max. 400 kcal total for whole meal) ✓

OR
■ Lamb Medallions with Blackcurrant Sauce (see recipe, p.248) served with 100g boiled new potatoes (with skins) and unlimited vegetables

Dessert
■ 1 Marks & Spencer meringue basket filled with 1 tsp 0% fat Greek yogurt and topped with 3 sliced strawberries ☑

Alcohol or high-fat treat
■ 50ml measure of any spirit plus a Slimline mixer
OR
■ 1 fun-size Twix

FIVE-MINUTE TONE-UP

See www.rosemaryconley.tv/ailpDay16

AEROBIC CHALLENGE

Power walk for 30 minutes, swinging your bent arms as you walk. Increase the pace now that you are slimmer and fitter!

Exercise tip
What activities or sport did you enjoy doing at school? What were you good at? Can you find someone to participate in a similar activity with you now? The key to fitness success is finding a form of exercise that you enjoy, because you are likely to do it more often. Give it some thought today and search out that tennis or badminton racquet, buy a football, a skipping rope or a hula hoop!

MOTIVATIONAL THOUGHT FOR THE DAY

Following a low-fat, low-Gi, calorie-controlled eating plan means you won't be depositing unnecessary fat around your body. Combining this way of eating with regular exercise that tones you up as you slim down is not that difficult. It's a question of mindset and once you've followed this lifestyle for 28 days you will have acquired a new habit – one that will dramatically enhance your future health. If eating healthily and taking regular exercise becomes your new lifestyle, you will be making a priceless investment in your future. And you should never have to go on a diet later in life because you will be maintaining a healthy pattern of eating and activity every day as a matter of course.

The great thing about Rosemary Conley Diet and Fitness Clubs is that we offer a workout at every class, so members still have a reason for coming even after they have reached their goal weight. I still teach my own classes in Leicester and about 15 of my members have been coming along on a Monday evening for more than 20 years! For them it's a fun night out that helps them to stay focused on eating sensibly and staying fit. The result is they enjoy good health and fit bodies.

Day 17

Do you have a pedometer? If you do, wear it every day to check how active you are. Aim to achieve 10,000 steps a day, or at least 2000 more steps than your usual number, as this will help you to lose your excess weight and also to maintain it once you have achieved a healthy weight. Children should aim to do even more steps a day – about 15,000 – for good health. If you don't own a pedometer, check out www.rosemaryconley.com for an easy-to-use version that is cheap and effective. I find wearing a pedometer extremely motivating as it encourages me to move about more.

Are you still doing well on the diet? If you find yourself feeling really peckish, rather than eating something you'll regret later, nibble on some chopped carrots and celery sprinkled with celery salt and have a low-calorie drink. Sometimes feelings of hunger can be confused with thirst.

Today's toning exercises work the abdominals, back muscles, thighs, shoulders, chest and underarms. When you work out with me on www.rosemaryconley.tv/ailpDay17 you will realise that we are now increasing the level of physical challenge to make the workout even more effective.

MENU

Breakfast
▨ 1 small banana, sliced, mixed with 115g sliced strawberries and 1 × 100g pot low-fat yogurt, any flavour (max. 100 kcal and 5% fat) ☑

Mid-morning power snack
▨ 5 mini low-fat bread sticks plus 1 tsp 0% fat Greek yogurt mixed with chopped chives ☑

Lunch
▨ Spread 2 slices wholegrain bread with horseradish sauce or Hellmann's Extra Light Mayonnaise and make into a jumbo sandwich with 30g wafer thin beef, chicken or ham, plus salad vegetables
OR
▨ Bombay Rice (see recipe, p.263) served with salad ☑

Mid-afternoon power snack
▨ 1 red Portion Pot® (115g) raspberries plus 50g strawberries ☑

Dinner
▨ Chilli Prawn or Quorn Stir-Fry with Asparagus: Dry-fry ½ chopped red onion and ½ crushed garlic clove in a non-stick pan until soft. Add 50g sliced asparagus and either 100g uncooked, shelled prawns or Quorn pieces and continue cooking for 2–3 minutes. Pour in 1 × 75g pack chilli stir-fry sauce and stir well to coat the prawns and vegetables. Bring to the boil, then turn off the heat. Serve with salad and garnish with fresh chives ☑ P

OR
- 1 × 300g pack Rosemary Conley Solo Slim Low-Fat Beef Meatballs and Potato (order from www.rosemaryconley.com) served with 100g vegetables of your choice (excluding potatoes).

Dessert
- 1 Marks & Spencer meringue nest filled with 1 tbsp 0% fat Greek yogurt and topped with 1 tbsp fresh raspberries or blueberries ☑

Alcohol or high-fat treat
- 75ml measure of sweet sherry
OR
- 1 × 19g bag Cheese & Onion Flavour Pom-Bear Teddy-shaped Potato Snacks ☑

FIVE-MINUTE TONE-UP

See www.rosemaryconley.tv/ailpDay17

AEROBIC CHALLENGE

If you have a skipping rope, try skipping for as long as you can. March on the spot to give you a chance to get your breath back, then skip some more!

Exercise tip
Make it a rule never to leave items at the bottom of your stairs to take up later. Each trip upstairs will help you to burn extra calories.

MOTIVATIONAL THOUGHT FOR THE DAY

By the time you reach Day 28 you will have developed the habit of eating low-fat, low-Gi foods and being more active in your everyday life. You will automatically choose the stairs in preference to the lift, and leaving the car behind occasionally and walking for those short errands will be second nature. That is what is so brilliant about this 28-day programme. It isn't just a get-slim-quick package, but a lifestyle change programme that can last a lifetime. After you have finished the initial 28 days, if you go back to eating the way you used to, you will regain the weight you have lost. So I really hope this easy way of eating and increased everyday activity becomes a way of life for you so you stay slim and fit for good.

Day 18

One of the benefits of this diet is that every breakfast is interchangeable with every other breakfast in the book. Same with the lunches and also the dinners. There is no need for you to eat anything you don't like or that doesn't fit in with your family's needs. However, it is worth trying new vegetables and other foods that you may not have eaten before. You might be in for some tasty surprises.

Today's toning exercises will trim your waist, strengthen your back and tone your backside, inner thighs and shoulders. Just log on to www.rosemaryconley.tv/ailpDay18 and we'll work out together.

MENU

Breakfast
■ 1 blue Portion Pot® (35g) uncooked porridge oats, cooked in water with 10 sultanas and served with milk from allowance ☑

Mid-morning power snack
■ 1 Asda Good For You Chicken Noodle Cup Soup

Lunch
■ Stir-Fry Chicken with Ginger: Chop 100g chicken breast (no skin) into bite-sized pieces and dry-fry in a non-stick pan with ½ crushed garlic clove. When the chicken has changed colour and is almost cooked through, add 1 chopped red or green pepper, 1 chopped celery stick, ½ chopped red onion, 25g mushrooms and 50g mangetout and dry-fry quickly but do not overcook. Just before serving add 1 tsp grated fresh ginger, soy sauce to taste and fresh coriander and heat through ⒫
OR
■ 1 × 175g oven-baked sweet potato topped with 75g baked beans and served with a side salad tossed in low-fat dressing of your choice ☑

Mid-afternoon power snack
■ 75g fresh mango ☑

Dinner
■ 1 × 115g salmon steak (raw weight), steamed or microwaved, served with 80g boiled new potatoes (with skins), 1 yellow Portion Pot® (70g) peas, plus 100g broccoli or asparagus and 1 tbsp Hellmann's Extra Light Mayonnaise
OR

■ Any low-fat vegetarian ready meal (max. 400 kcal and 5 % fat, including any accompaniments) ✓

Dessert
■ 1 × 120g pot Danone Shape Fat Free Feel Fuller For Longer yogurt, any flavour ✓

Alcohol or high-fat treat
■ 100ml measure of Martini Extra Dry plus Slimline mixer
OR
■ 2 Weight Watchers Double Choc Chip Cookies ✓

FIVE-MINUTE TONE-UP

See www.rosemaryconley.tv/ailpDay18

AEROBIC CHALLENGE

Walk up and down stairs 5 times consecutively, then repeat later in the day. In addition, go for a 15-minute brisk walk or work out at a class or to a fitness DVD.

> **Exercise tip**
> Did you know that working as a chambermaid is one of the most active jobs you can do? It burns more calories than most other occupations because chambermaids are on their feet most of the day and use quite a bit of strength making beds and so on. So, next time you make your bed and do the housework, remember that you are burning calories and, instead of seeing it as a chore, think of it as a workout and do it with extra zeal.

MOTIVATIONAL THOUGHT FOR THE DAY

After today there are only ten days to go before you complete the 28-day programme. What a fantastic achievement that will be and think of how much slimmer you will look and feel compared to when you started the programme. It's difficult to predict the exact rate at which we will lose weight. Sometimes the scales tell us we haven't lost much yet the tape measure shows that we are definitely losing inches. That's why it's worth taking the time to measure yourself once a week so you don't lose heart. All you can do is give it your best effort – so stick to the diet, do the exercises and activities as described and continue to be as active as you can every day. The results will be phenomenal and you will be so pleased you made the effort.

Day 19

Ten days to go and everything to look forward to. Your body is getting used to being fed a healthy diet of smaller quantities of food than previously as well as benefiting from increased levels of activity, and you are reaping the rewards. It's as if your body is giving a huge sigh of relief and thinking 'At last I'm being fed what I need to be healthy!'

It can be quite frightening to realise how much we have abused our bodies over the years and how, despite the bad treatment, they have somehow managed to survive and support us. But only now will you be enjoying the full extent of the benefits of eating a much healthier diet and using your muscles more.

Muscles respond wonderfully to being used and challenged, and exercise is our passport to a longer, more independent, life. There is no downside, providing you are wise about the amount of exercise you do and you listen to your body so you know when you've done enough. Try your best to complete today's toning exercises, which focus on the abdominals, outer thighs and front thighs, chest, underarms and shoulders.

Start enjoying that looser waistband and the extra energy you will be experiencing. Have a good day.

MENU

Breakfast
- 1 yellow Portion Pot® (14 Minis) Weetabix Fruit 'n' Nut Minis, plus 1 medium-sized banana, sliced, served with milk from allowance ☑

Mid-morning power snack
- 12 seedless grapes ☑

Lunch
- 1 medium slice wholegrain bread, toasted, topped with 1 × 125g can sardines or mackerel fillets, plus a small salad
OR
- 1 can any lentil or bean soup (max. 250 kcal and 5% fat), plus 1 piece fresh fruit (excluding bananas) ☑

Mid-afternoon power snack
- 10 sweet silverskin pickled onions plus 10 cherry tomatoes ☑

Dinner
- Chicken or Quorn in Mushroom Sauce: Dry-fry 100g chopped chicken breast (no skin) or Quorn alternative with ½ chopped onion and 6 button mushrooms. When the chicken is almost cooked, add 100g (⅓ can) Batchelors Low Fat Condensed Mushroom Soup, plus milk from allowance if needed to make a creamy sauce. Simmer until the chicken is completely cooked. Serve with 1 yellow Portion Pot® (100g) mashed sweet potato, plus other vegetables of your choice ☑
OR
- 1 × 300g pack Rosemary Conley Solo Slim Lamb Hotpot (order from www.rosemaryconley.com) served with 100g new potatoes (with skins) plus 100g green vegetables of your choice

Dessert
- 1 × 55g pot Asda Great Fruity Stuff fromage frais, any flavour ☑

Alcohol or high-fat treat
- 300ml (½ pint) dry cider

OR
- 1 × 23g bag Walkers French Fries Ready Salted crisps ☑

FIVE-MINUTE TONE-UP

See www.rosemaryconley.tv/ailpDay19

AEROBIC CHALLENGE

Go for a 20-minute brisk walk, then skip for 5 minutes (if you have a skipping rope). To finish, march on the spot for 2 minutes to cool down. Don't forget to do your stretches.

Exercise tip

You could increase your daily calorie output by as much as 200 extra calories just by making some small changes to your everyday routine. By using the stairs instead of the lift, parking your car further away or getting off the bus a stop earlier, walking to your colleague's desk to ask a question rather than phoning or e-mailing, standing up to make phone calls, taking a walk at lunchtime or going shopping and carrying the bags – all manner of little extras that mount up and burn extra calories.

MOTIVATIONAL THOUGHT FOR THE DAY

The fact that you have reached this exciting stage of your weight loss journey is very significant. The first two weeks were tough, but you managed. You are now five days into the second phase of this Amazing Inch Loss Plan and, despite having a couple of hundred extra calories to spend each day, your body is now in serious fat-burning mode. Your daily activity is being fuelled entirely from your fat stores and all the calories you are eating are being spent by your body to keep it functioning healthily.

Your body is being given five-star fuel, because everything you are eating is healthy, and your body is happy because it is in training to become fitter and to function at optimum efficiency. Our bodies were not designed to spend most of the day sitting behind a desk, in front of a computer, a steering wheel or a television. Our ancestors walked everywhere and spent most of the day outside, tending the land and growing their own food.

Should you get any hunger pangs, look upon this as a sign that your body is in calorie-deficit and you are getting slimmer by the day! If you feel really hungry between meals, have a low-calorie drink and nibble on some chopped vegetables. I know these are not as exciting as a packet of crisps but at least they won't make you fat.

Day 20

The exercises that I'm teaching you each day on www.rosemaryconley.tv are becoming much more challenging now. Please try your best to do them, but if you find any of them too hard, just do the easier versions that I show you and then progress at a level that you feel is right for you. When you reach the end of the 28-day programme, I suggest you return to Day 14 (www.rosemaryconley.tv/ailpDay14) and repeat the last two weeks of the exercise programme, always doing the advanced versions of the individual toning exercises. If you are able to do them every day you will be astonished at how fast you will progress. But it's a myth to think that you have to be an exercise junkie to have a good body. Absolutely not. Once you have lost your unwanted weight, you can keep in great shape by doing a variety of exercises on a fairly regular basis.

Today's toning exercises work the abdominals, back and shoulders and hips. Once you master these more challenging moves, you will be able to work your muscles very effectively in a short period of time.

MENU

Breakfast
Mix 100g 0% fat Greek yogurt with 1 blue Portion Pot®
(40g) muesli and a little semi-skimmed milk from allowance to
moisten. Add a little Silver Spoon Half Spoon to sweeten to
taste. Leave to soak overnight in the refrigerator for best
results. Serve chilled ☑

Mid-morning power snack
100g fresh pineapple ☑

Lunch
Tuna or Chicken Pasta Salad: 1 red Portion Pot® (110g
cooked weight) pasta shapes mixed with either 50g drained
canned tuna (in brine) or 30g chopped cooked chicken breast,
plus unlimited chopped peppers, red onion, cucumber, tomato
and celery and 2 tsps Hellmann's Extra Light Mayonnaise or
low-fat thousand island dressing
OR
Any pre-packed sandwich (max. 300 kcal and 5% fat) ☑

Mid-afternoon power snack
20g low-fat cheese (max. 5% fat) plus 5 cherry tomatoes ☑

Dinner
150g tuna steak, grilled, served with 1 blue Portion Pot®
(50g uncooked weight) couscous (any flavour, e.g. see Ainsley
Harriott range) plus 1 blue Portion Pot® (75g) tomato salsa
and a large salad
OR

■ Roasted Pepper Pasta (see recipe, p.261) served with a large salad and low-fat dressing ✓

Dessert
■ Eton Mess: Break up 1 Marks & Spencer meringue basket and mix with 1 tbsp 0% fat Greek yogurt and 1 large strawberry, chopped ✓

Alcohol or high-fat treat
■ 75ml Martini Rosso plus a low-calorie mixer
OR
■ 2 Galaxy Mini Eggs ✓

FIVE-MINUTE TONE-UP

See www.rosemaryconley.tv/ailpDay20

AEROBIC CHALLENGE

Work out energetically to a fitness DVD for 30 minutes or go for a 30-minute brisk walk.

Exercise tip

Next time you arrange to meet friends socially, why not suggest doing something active like ten pin bowling or ice skating or dancing. They are all great fun and much healthier than just sitting down eating and drinking all evening.

MOTIVATIONAL THOUGHT FOR THE DAY

Eating is an enjoyable habit but sometimes we can drift back into the old habits that made us overweight in the first place. We all have our favourite foods and it's fine to eat them occasionally, but only if we can trust ourselves not to eat them every day.

Eating big portions is another habit we can fall into. It is easy to convince ourselves that we are eating the correct amount of food, and staying within our daily calorie allowance, but often we are deceiving ourselves. Studies have shown that people tend to underestimate the quantity of food they eat and overestimate how active they are. That's why following a plan like this one, where the calories are controlled and the exercises are specific, is so effective. So weigh out your portions (or use my Portion Pots®) to avoid disappointment on the scales. If you allow yourself that extra shake of cereal from the packet, that extra half tablespoon of boiled rice and curry and that extra glass of wine or orange juice, it really can affect your progress. So, in the run up to the last few days on this plan, make a massive effort to stick to the quantities given and to do the recommended activities. You will be grateful in the long run when you see the benefits.

Day 21

This is the final day of week three and it's your third weigh-in day tomorrow, so it's crucial you try to achieve as positive a response as possible on the scales. Be strict with your portion sizes, weighing out or measuring all your servings of food. Try to keep busy today so your mind is fully occupied and you are not constantly thinking about food. I also recommend you don't have any alcohol today as it can make you dehydrated and cause you to drink extra fluid to compensate, though I am in no way suggesting that you cut back on fluids. It is really important that you stay hydrated. You want to lose fat, not water.

Today is an aerobic day so there are no toning exercises, but aim to do as much aerobic activity as you can fit into your schedule as I really want you to keep moving as much as possible and burn lots of calories. Really go for it today.

MENU

Breakfast
- 2 turkey rashers and 1 low-fat beef or pork sausage (max. 5% fat), grilled or dry-fried, served with 1 × 200g can tomatoes boiled until reduced and 100g grilled mushrooms **P**
OR
- 2 Quorn sausages, grilled, served with 1 × 400g can tomatoes boiled until reduced, plus 50g grilled mushrooms **V**

Mid-morning power snack
- 1 × 200g slice melon (weighed without skin) **V**

Lunch
- Large mixed salad plus 1 smoked mackerel fillet or 1 × 125g can sardines or salmon (not in oil), served with 2 tsps Hellmann's Extra Light Mayonnaise or other low-fat dressing of your choice. Plus 1 pear or orange **P**
OR
- Chicken, Mushroom and Lemon Soup (see recipe, p.241) served with a small wholegrain roll (max. 150 kcal). Plus 1 pear or orange

Mid-afternoon power snack
- 150g strawberries **V**

Dinner
- 100g lean roast beef, thinly sliced, served with 100g dry-roasted potatoes and 200g other vegetables of your choice (excluding potatoes), plus low-fat gravy and 1 tsp horseradish sauce
OR

- Sweet and Sour Quorn: Dry-fry ½ pack (175g) of Quorn Chicken Style Pieces with ½ chopped onion, ½ chopped red and green pepper, 5 button mushrooms, halved, 1 chopped celery stick, 1 small courgette, halved and chopped, ½ pack of fresh (or 1 whole can) beansprouts. Do not overcook. Add 1 yellow Portion Pot® (125ml) Uncle Ben's Sweet & Sour Light sauce and heat through before serving ☑P

Plus 1 low-fat yogurt (max. 100 kcal and 5% fat) in addition to dessert below

Dessert
- 1 Asda Good For You Lemon Slice ☑

Alcohol or high-fat treat
- 300ml (½ pint) Guinness

OR

- 1 Thorntons Mini Caramel Shortcake ☑

FIVE-MINUTE TONE-UP

Rest day.

AEROBIC CHALLENGE

Try and work out for an hour today. Salsacise, aerobics, a class, swimming energetically, working out to a DVD, using cardio equipment at the gym – they all use extra calories and they all burn fat. Drink plenty of water before, during and after your workout.

Exercise tip

Washing the car is an excellent workout. It involves quite a lot of energy and strength to clean and polish the paintwork before it dries to prevent those ugly smears. See your car washing as a workout and do it more often.

MOTIVATIONAL THOUGHT FOR THE DAY

Try to make a special effort with your appearance today and wear something that shows you have lost weight. Ladies, put on some make-up, style your hair carefully and wear some pretty jewellery. Gentlemen, wear something different that fits you well, and try to look super-smart today.

If someone compliments you on your appearance, accept the compliment with good grace. Thank the person and say: 'That's really encouraging. I am trying very hard to lose weight at the moment.' Often when someone pays us a compliment we get embarrassed and throw it back at them by saying something like: 'Well yes, I've lost a bit, but I'm still huge.' You can be pretty sure that the person who made the kind comment won't venture there again!

So, make a conscious decision that if someone does make a flattering comment you will enjoy it and be ready with your gracious response.

Day 22

Today is your third weighing and measuring day. This third weigh-in is perhaps the hardest to face, as you have increased your calories a little over the last week and your body has now got used to eating fewer calories than it was receiving up to three weeks ago. As a result, you may not see the same level of weight loss on the scales as you did at the end of week two. This is to be expected, so please don't be discouraged.

You are probably finding you get a bit hungry more often – but remember, this is great news as it shows your body is having to draw on your energy stores of fat distributed around your body to make up the shortfall. Also, you might be finding that your energy levels are flagging a little, as your body is now in full fat-burning mode. I can only promise you that it will get easier and you only have one week to go at this lower calorie level (unless you are over 60 or very slim!). I've given you a rest day from aerobic exercise today, and the five-minute tone-up is quick to do and doesn't use too much energy, yet it is extremely effective. Log on to www.rosemaryconley.tv /ailpDay22 for today's exercises, which work the abdominals and back, the outer thighs, and the chest and underarm muscles. Just stick with it and trust me that the results in a week's time will be worth it.

MENU

Breakfast
▤ 2 Weetabix served with milk from allowance and 2 tsps sugar or 1 mini banana ☑

Mid-morning power snack
▤ 1 small apple ☑

Lunch
▤ 1 × 40g granary baguette spread with 20g Philadelphia Extra Light soft cheese then topped with 25g wafer thin ham or Quorn Deli Ham Style, 1 sliced tomato and mustard to taste, plus a small side salad ☑

Mid-afternoon power snack
▤ 1 Rakusen's cracker topped with 1 × 20g triangle Laughing Cow Extra Light soft cheese, plus 5 cherry tomatoes

Dinner
▤ Fish Pie: Place 50g each of fresh salmon, cod and shelled uncooked prawns in a small ovenproof dish and cover with ⅓ can Batchelors Low Fat Condensed Mushroom Soup, top with mashed potato (made by boiling 115g old potatoes then mashing with milk from allowance and seasoning well). Place in the oven and bake at 200C, 400F, Gas Mark 6 for 30 minutes or until the potato is browned on top. Serve with unlimited carrots and broccoli ℗
OR
▤ Quorn and Rice Bake (see recipe, p.262) served with unlimited vegetables (excluding potatoes) ☑

Dessert
- 1 × 70g pot Marks & Spencer Count On Us Raspberry Mousse

Alcohol or high-fat treat
- 1 yellow Portion Pot® (125ml) red or white wine
OR
- 1 McVitie's Belgian Chocolate Chunk Boaster ☑

FIVE-MINUTE TONE-UP

See www.rosemaryconley.tv/ailpDay22

AEROBIC CHALLENGE

Rest day.

Exercise tip

Try balancing on one leg when you are cleaning your teeth or talking on the phone. This might sound odd, but it will help to improve your balance as well as your posture. Balance is something we can learn at any age and it helps us to stay safe as we are less likely to fall over. It is particularly helpful for mature folk to practise this.

MOTIVATIONAL THOUGHT FOR THE DAY

When you got on the scales this morning, if you found you hadn't lost the half stone you felt you deserved to have lost this week because you have been so good, don't despair. Measure yourself and see for yourself that lots of inches have in fact disappeared this week and that is what matters. You are getting slimmer. People are noticing and your clothes are looser.

The mid-morning and mid-afternoon power snacks are there to help you stave off hunger pangs, so make sure you eat them. It's important that you don't eat less food than is recommended in the eating plan. And are you drinking enough fluids? Sometimes our energy levels can plummet if we get dehydrated, so drink plenty of water, weak tea or low-calorie drinks to keep your fluid levels adequately topped up.

I hope you enjoy your toning exercises today. As your muscles are now stronger, you will be able to do these more advanced moves and reap the benefits to your body shape. And the aerobic challenge will help you to burn more body fat, so do your best to fit it in. You are winning the weight loss battle and the rewards are huge.

Day 23

Now you are well into week four, take time to appreciate your monumental achievements so far. Your body is getting used to eating healthier food, doing lots of different exercises and will be feeling slimmer and fitter. What are the things you have noticed most? Are you finding it easier to fit into the bath? Do you no longer get so out of breath when you go upstairs? Are your clothes feeling looser and more comfortable rather than feeling as if they are 'strangling' you? No doubt you are experiencing enormous benefits all round.

The daily exercises are becoming increasingly challenging as each day progresses, so listen to your body and only do what you feel you can manage. Today we are using a chair again and the workout includes exercises for the stomach, backside, inner and front thighs as well as the underarms. The harder the exercises become, the more effective they will be at strengthening and shaping your muscles. And the stronger your muscles, the greater the amount of fat that will be burnt in them when you do your aerobic exercises. Be encouraged. You are really doing the business now and your body is undergoing a significant transformation.

MENU

Breakfast
▦ ½ fresh grapefruit plus 2 medium-sized boiled eggs ☑️🅿️

Mid-morning power snack
▦ 1 blue Portion Pot® (75g) tomato salsa, plus 1 carrot,
1 celery stick and 1 × 5cm piece cucumber sliced into
crudités ☑️

Lunch
▦ Chicken and Rice Salad: 80g (cooked weight) boiled basmati
rice mixed with 60g cooked chopped chicken breast (no skin),
chopped peppers, red onion, mushrooms, celery and 1 tbsp
sweetcorn kernels. Season with freshly ground black pepper
and soy sauce or fat-free dressing of your choice
OR
▦ Singapore Noodles with Prawns (see recipe, p.257) plus a
crisp salad

Mid-afternoon power snack
▦ 1 fat-free yogurt (max. 50 kcal) ☑️

Dinner
▦ Baked Liver and Onions: Place 150g calves' liver in an
ovenproof dish with 1 sliced onion. Cover with foil and cook in
a moderate oven (180C, 350F, Gas Mark 4) for 15–20 minutes
until lightly cooked. Make some low-fat gravy with gravy
powder and add to the liver and onion. Serve with 1 yellow
Portion Pot® (100g) mashed potato and other vegetables of
your choice
OR

- Cheesy Cottage Pie (see recipe, p.249)

Dessert
- Tropical Sorbet (see recipe, p.267) ☑

Alcohol or high-fat treat
- 300ml (½ pint) lager or beer
OR
- 1 Kellogg's Coco Pops Cereal & Milk Bar ☑

FIVE-MINUTE TONE-UP

See www.rosemaryconley.tv/ailpDay23

AEROBIC CHALLENGE

Work out at an aerobics class or do a fitness DVD for 40 minutes, or go for a 40-minute brisk walk, or jog for 20 minutes or walk up and down stairs 5 times consecutively and repeat 3 times throughout the day.

Exercise tip

If you have a small trampoline or any piece of home gym equipment, why not get it out of the loft or the garage, dust it off and have a go on it. Put on some lively music and bounce, pedal, row or run on it. Exercise can be monotonous sometimes and if we vary our activities, we are more likely to keep it up.

MOTIVATIONAL THOUGHT FOR THE DAY

If we are to succeed at anything – and that includes losing weight and getting fitter – it's crucial that we are motivated by the end goal, and the rewards that we enjoy along the way will help us to reach that goal.

Rewards are very motivating and at least 50 per cent of the pleasure is the 'looking forward to it' bit. So, decide what you would like as a reward for each stone you lose or for when your weight enters a new weight-bracket (such as getting to 12 stone-something from being 13 stone-something) and then decide on an ultimate reward for when you reach your goal weight.

If you have a generous and supportive partner, maybe they could sponsor you for each pound or stone you lose so that you can treat yourself to some lovely new clothes when you reach your goal. Or perhaps you dream of having a makeover or going to a health spa for a weekend or even just for a day. You choose, but discuss it with the family so that they know where you are aiming and they can encourage you and enjoy the journey with you.

Start planning a reward for your efforts this week, even if you don't actually receive the reward until some time in the future. If you have to wait, you can enjoy the looking-forward-to-it bit all the more!

Day 24

As you move towards the end of the 28-day programme, really step up your efforts with the exercise plan. The more challenging the exercises become, the more effective they will be.

Today's toning exercises work the abdominals, back and shoulders, and outer thighs. Try to perform them to the best of your ability as you work out with me on www.rosemaryconley.tv/ailpDay24 and feel the action of each muscle as it works hard. Focus on that feeling in the muscle to help maximise the effect of the exercise and also to make sure you are doing the exercise correctly. If you can't feel anything happening to the muscle, probably not much will be happening!

Your aerobic fitness should have improved significantly by now. Try to walk a bit faster and jog for longer if you can. If jogging proves too difficult for you, because of pressure on your knees or hips, then try power walking, which is just as effective providing you don't mind keeping going for a little longer to cover the same distance. Both jogging and power walking are fantastic fat burners.

MENU

Breakfast
■ 200g fresh fruit salad topped with 100g Total 2 % fat Greek Yoghurt and 6 sultanas ☑

Mid-morning power snack
■ 10 cherry tomatoes, plus chunks of carrots, cucumber and green or red pepper ☑

Lunch
■ 1 bagel cut in half, spread with 20g Philadelphia Extra Light soft cheese then topped with 50g smoked salmon and freshly ground black pepper or chopped fresh dill
OR
■ 1 × 50g wholemeal pitta bread filled with 50g low-fat houmous and chopped mixed salad sprinkled with low-fat dressing of your choice ☑

Mid-afternoon power snack
■ 2 satsumas ☑

Dinner
■ Steak in Mushroom Sauce: Dry-fry 2 thin beef steaks (250g total) or 2 Quorn Peppered Steaks quickly on both sides. Remove from the pan and keep warm. Add 100g chestnut mushrooms to the pan and cook for 1 minute before adding 1 tsp Knorr Touch of Taste beef stock (or vegetarian alternative) and 75ml water. Bring the sauce to the boil and reduce by half. Remove from the heat and stir in ½ tbsp 3 % fat yogurt. Transfer the steaks to serving plates and top with the mushroom sauce. Serve with green vegetables or salad ☑ P

OR

■ Chinese Chicken Kebabs (see recipe, p.243) served with 1 blue Portion Pot® (55g uncooked weight) or 1 red Portion Pot® (144g cooked weight) basmati rice per person

Dessert
■ 1 × 70g pot Marks & Spencer Count On Us Chocolate Mousse

Alcohol or high-fat treat
■ 50ml measure of port
OR
■ 1 Green & Black's Organic Chocolate Flapjack biscuit ☑

FIVE-MINUTE TONE-UP

See www.rosemaryconley.tv/ailpDay24

AEROBIC CHALLENGE

Go for a power walk and intersperse some jogging steps even if you manage only 20 or so. Try to keep going for 30 minutes.

Exercise tip

Did you know that dog walkers are on average a stone lighter than non-dog owners? Dog walking is a great way to burn extra calories. It works because the dog provides the purpose for the excursion and the motivation to put on your walking shoes. As one doctor told me: 'The NHS should provide everyone with a dog – it would transform their health!' If you don't have a dog of your own, maybe you could borrow one from a friend or neighbour?

MOTIVATIONAL THOUGHT FOR THE DAY

Just four days to go after today and then you can calculate how many calories you are allowed on the third phase of this Amazing Inch Loss Plan in order to lose the rest of your unwanted weight. The heavier you are, the more calories you will be allowed and if you are young, you will be surprised at how many you can have.

As we get older we burn fewer calories, so we have to accept that we must eat less if we are to avoid weight gain. We tend not to be as active as we were in our twenties and so sometimes, thankfully, our appetite will decrease too. Mine certainly did as I reached my late fifties and early sixties and I now find that I can get halfway through a meal and my stomach says: 'That's it! I don't want any more.' I don't fight it. I'm just really glad that my appestat (the bit of our brain that tells us when we've eaten enough) is working at last!

Over the last three-and-a-half weeks you have re-educated your appetite, your palate and your eating habits, and the changes you have made will have turned your body into a highly efficient machine. Your blood pressure and your cholesterol levels will be healthier, your muscles will have become stronger and your organs – liver, kidneys, etc. – will feel like they've had a holiday as they won't have had to work so hard processing all the high-fat food you ate previously. By the end of this week you will have given your body the equivalent of a 50,000-mile service and it will be feeling terrific.

Day 25

Are you still sticking strictly to the diet? It's important that you still keep tabs on what you are eating and don't become too relaxed. Adding an extra slice of ham to your sandwich ('to finish off the packet'), or eating a couple of sweets offered by colleagues and finishing those leftovers on the children's plates are all pitfalls to which we can easily succumb, and the cumulative value of the extra calories in a day could easily be 500! Over a week that would amount to one pound of body fat and the spoiling of your weight loss progress. So be extra-vigilant over these last few days and be as active as you possibly can. 'Walk more, drive less' is this week's motto!

Today's toning exercises are even more challenging, but as we work out together on www.rosemaryconley.tv/ailpDay25 I will talk you through them and show alternatives. As you become fitter and stronger you will be able to progress to these advanced moves. Today we are working the stomach, back, backside, legs and shoulders. Do your best.

MENU

Breakfast
■ ½ bagel (or 1 whole mini bagel) toasted, spread with 1 tsp fruit preserve, jam, honey or marmalade then topped with 50g 2% fat Total Greek Yoghurt ✓

Mid-morning power snack
- 1 kid's fun-size mini banana ☑

Lunch
- 75g cooked egg noodles tossed with unlimited beansprouts, spring onions, chopped peppers, fresh coriander and 75g flaked cooked salmon, served with soy sauce
OR
- Cheese and Marmite Sandwich: Spread 2 slices wholegrain bread with Marmite and fill with 40g low-fat cottage cheese ☑

Mid-afternoon power snack
- 1 kiwi fruit plus 5 seedless grapes ☑

Dinner
- Beef Fajitas: Dry-fry 120g sliced lean beef with ½ each sliced red and green pepper and ½ chopped red onion, then mix in 2 tsps fajita spice mix. Fill a low-fat tortilla wrap with the mixture and serve with 1 blue Portion Pot® (75g) tomato salsa and a large mixed salad tossed in oil-free dressing
OR
- Chicken Shaslik (see recipe, p.245) served with 1 blue Portion Pot® (55g uncooked weight) or 1 red Portion Pot® (144g cooked weight) basmati rice per person

Dessert
- 1 × 200g pot Müllerlight Wild Blueberry fat free yogurt

Alcohol or high-fat treat
- 1 blue Portion Pot® (80ml) dry sherry
OR
- 6 Cadbury Mini Eggs ☑

FIVE-MINUTE TONE-UP

See www.rosemaryconley.tv/ailpDay25

AEROBIC CHALLENGE

Go swimming, cycling, jogging, or anything that causes you to become mildly breathless. Try and work out for 30 minutes and remember to do your stretches at the end (see pp.343–7).

Exercise tip

Research has shown that couples are more likely to enjoy greater success on a first date if they do something active, e.g. a game of sport, walking or dancing, rather than having a passive evening watching a film or dining out. The physical activity acts as an alternative focal point and we can learn a lot about the other person when interacting in this way.

MOTIVATIONAL THOUGHT FOR THE DAY

We often say we don't have time to exercise, yet in the UK we watch an average of three hours of television a day!

I believe the main reason we don't exercise as much as we should is that many of us don't find a form of exercise that we really enjoy. We can buy the latest hi-tech exercise bike/treadmill/rowing machine, but after the first flurry of activity, it tends to be demoted to the garage, loft, spare bedroom or used as a clothes horse. Why? Because many people find them deadly boring! Men are much more likely to increase their fitness by playing a sport such as tennis, golf, badminton or squash – sports that are competitive, fun and also great workouts. Some people love swimming and can swim up to 40 lengths at a time. And the reason many people enjoy working out to a fitness DVD or attending an aerobics class is that they have to use their brains as well as their bodies to coordinate the moves. This is both stimulating and interesting and means they don't get bored.

During this four-week programme I have given you a specific exercise challenge each day and, because each day's challenge is different and gets more demanding as you progress, it becomes interesting as well as, hopefully, rewarding. At the end of this week you will need to decide what activity you are going to do on an ongoing basis.

Attending a Rosemary Conley Diet and Fitness Club class is one of the best things you could do as you will be personally supervised to ensure you do the exercises correctly. The workouts at these classes, and in any of my DVDs, use all the muscles in the body and provides an efficient all-round fitness training activity that incorporates fat burning and body toning exercises as well as a stretch session to increase flexibility. Add some regular brisk walking and perhaps an active sport or hobby, and you will be doing sufficient activity to help you continue to lose weight and maintain your new weight and your figure long term.

Day 26

Just three days to go – three crucial days until the end of this 28-day marathon! If you are still with me, I am so proud of you and you will be thrilled with the end results. However, you will need to be prepared for temptation to come knocking at your door at some point in the future to tease you away from your successful challenge. So put on your metaphorical bullet-proof vest and the arrows of temptation will just bounce off you and you will stay focused.

Plan to have a celebratory meal on Day 29 and treat yourself to some champagne. You will thoroughly deserve it. But for now, stick to the diet and be as active as you can. There are no toning exercises today, so give today's aerobic challenge your best effort. Enjoy your day!

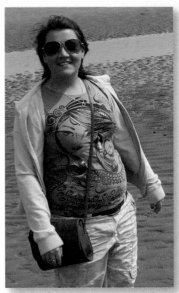

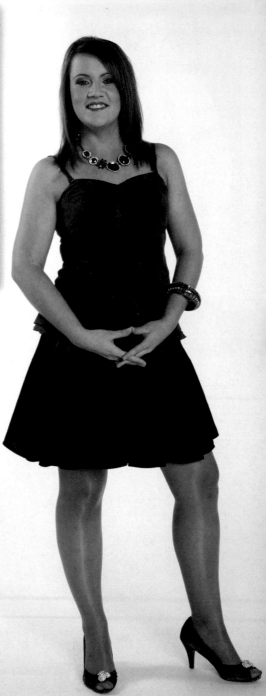

'The Amazing Inch Loss Plan is my life now, I don't even have to think about it.'
Jane Gillespie

Trialist Jane lost 1st 7lb in four weeks and went on to lose 2st 10lb in total

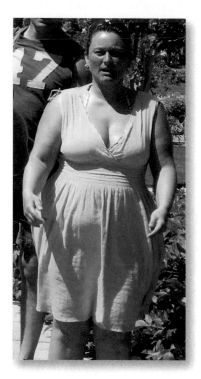

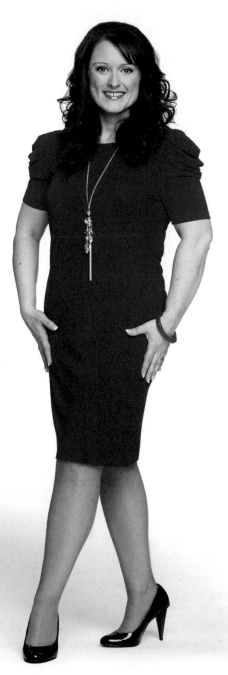

'I lost almost a stone in four weeks, but the biggest shock was my inch loss! I no longer suffer from heartburn or acid indigestion. I have more energy and can walk without getting out of breath. I can't believe how much food you can eat in one day!'
Jeanette Hopkins

Trialist Jeanette lost 13lb in four weeks and went on to lose 2st 5lb

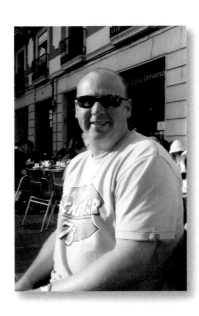

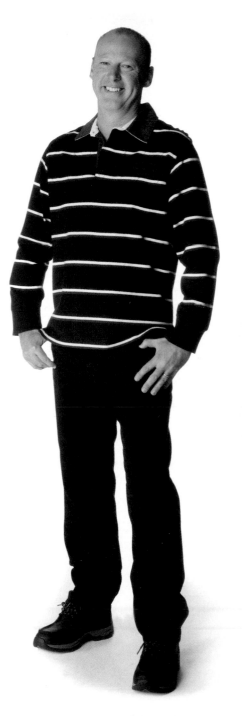

'I no longer have to take
tablets for cholesterol and
blood pressure and I have
to see the doctor only once
a year, instead of once
every two months.'
Andrew Corbett

Trialist Andrew lost 1st 8lb
in one month and went on
to lose a total of 3 stone

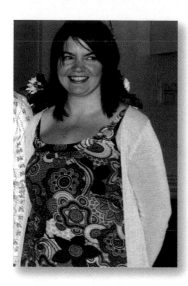

'I started to enjoy exercise
because it made a huge
difference to my weight
loss and toned up all of
the flabby bits.'
Teresa O'Neill

Trialist Teresa lost 11lb and
dropped two dress sizes in
four weeks

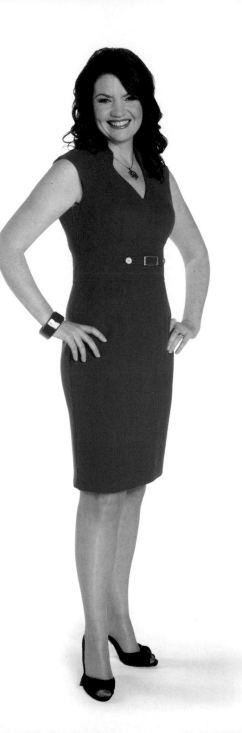

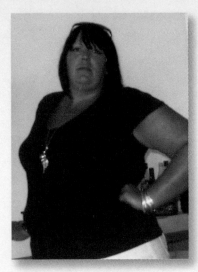

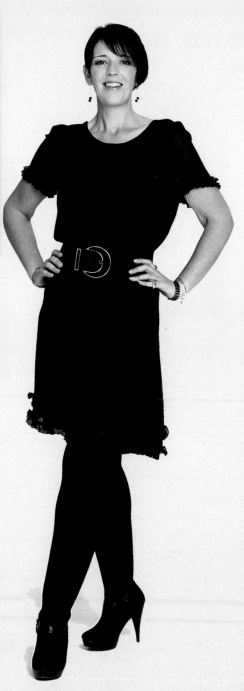

'I was shocked at how quickly I lost the weight and I'm still not used to the new me. It's the best thing I've ever done. It's been fantastic!'
Club member Stephanie Hughes

Stephanie lost 12 stone in 10 months on the Amazing Inch Loss Plan at her local Rosemary Conley class run by Rachel Burton

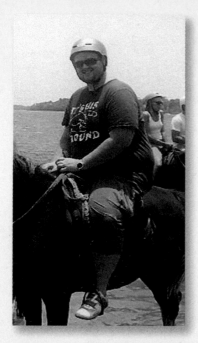

'The weight just fell off because I stuck to the diet – I couldn't believe it!'
Club member Michael Hutchinson

Michael lost 10 stone in 10 months on the Amazing Inch Loss Plan at his local Rosemary Conley class run by Carol Wilson

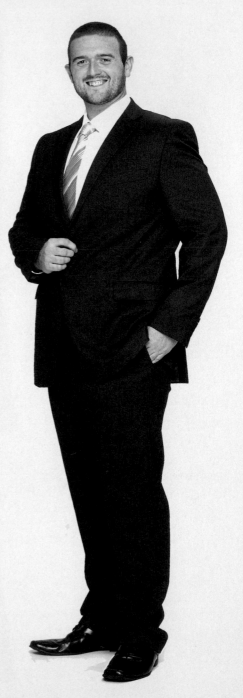

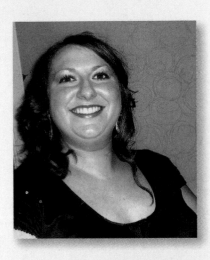

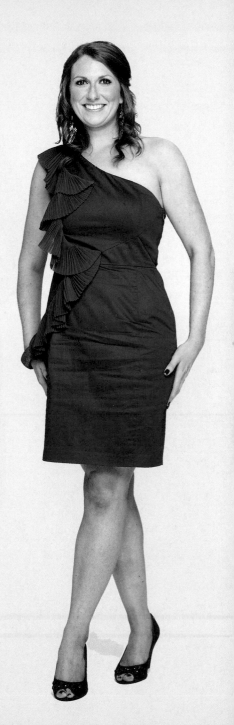

'The diet is easy to follow because everything is explained well and the classes are a great support. I feel brilliant – now I can shop wherever I want!'
Club member Eve Leonard

Twenty-two-year-old student Eve lost 5st 10lb in nine months at her local Rosemary Conley class run by Mandi Davidson

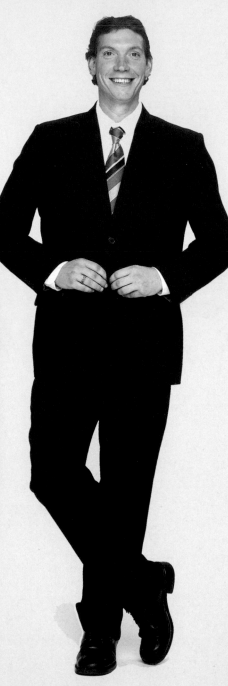

'I grabbed this diet by the horns and now I've done it I couldn't be happier. I lost 9st in six months'
Club member Carl Williams

Carl followed the Amazing Inch Loss Plan at his local Rosemary Conley class, which is run by Freda MacDonald

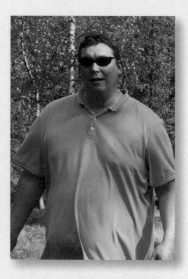

MENU

Breakfast

▨ 2 low-fat (max. 5 % fat) beef, pork or Quorn sausages, grilled, served with 1 yellow Portion Pot® (115g) baked beans and 50g grilled mushrooms ✓P

Mid-morning power snack

▨ 1 red Portion Pot® (115g) raspberries topped with 2 tsps low-fat yogurt (max. 5 % fat) ✓

Lunch

▨ 2-egg omelette made using milk from allowance and lots of freshly ground black pepper, and filled with chopped peppers, red onion, mushrooms and 25g grated low-fat cheese (max. 5 % fat) ✓P

Mid-afternoon power snack

▨ 1 Hartley's Low Calorie Jelly topped with 1 tbsp Total 2 % Greek Yoghurt and 3 berries of your choice

Dinner

▨ 175g lean beef fillet or rump steak or 2 Quorn Peppered Steaks, grilled, served with a large salad plus 1 tbsp Hellmann's Extra Light Mayonnaise ✓P
OR
▨ Cauliflower Bhaji (see recipe, p.265) served with 1 blue Portion Pot® (55g uncooked weight) or 1 red Portion Pot® (144g cooked weight) basmati rice per person ✓

Dessert

▨ 1 × 120g pot Del Monte Fruitini Fruit Pieces in juice ✓

Alcohol or high-fat treat

- 1 yellow Portion Pot® (125ml) red or white wine

OR

- 1 × 21g bag Boots Shapers Salt & Vinegar Chipsticks ☑

FIVE-MINUTE TONE-UP

Rest day.

AEROBIC CHALLENGE

Choose any physical activity you like that is going to make you slightly breathless but that you can sustain for 45 minutes.

Exercise tip

Having the right shoes and fitness gear can increase our motivation to exercise. They don't need to be exotic, just comfortable and flattering. Now that you are slimmer, why not treat yourself?

MOTIVATIONAL THOUGHT FOR THE DAY

Over the last four weeks you will have dropped at least one dress size, maybe two. Why not look for something new to wear on Day 29 that will show off your new, slimmer figure? Remember, if you have still a significant amount of excess weight to lose, have a look in a dress agency, where nearly-new clothes are sold at a fraction of the original cost, or in a charity shop where clothes can be had at bargain prices, to see if there is something that fits you for now and that you can recycle once you have lost more weight.

Plan to give yourself a mini-makeover on Day 29. Think about having your hair restyled, and perhaps having a professional make-up session – or at least treat yourself to some new products. If you make a real effort it will give you extra confidence and show the world that you are proud of what you have achieved over the last four weeks.

As these last few days creep up on you, it is good to keep your mind occupied with thoughts of these exciting treats rather than treats in the form of food!

Day 27

Only two days of the 28-day programme to go. For every day that you complete on this programme you are taking a very significant step towards your ultimate success because if you can give yourself the very best start to your weight-loss plan, you are much more likely to succeed in the long term. This four-week challenge – and no one is denying that it is challenging – provides you with a cracking start that will make a real difference to your health, your fitness and your size. So stay focused.

I have extended today's and tomorrow's toning sessions to cover more muscle groups so that by the end of tomorrow you will have worked the whole body with these very advanced exercises. Log on to www.rosemaryconley.tv/ailpDay27 and give them your best effort and realise how much stronger your muscles are now compared to when you started the programme. Do not falter! Be as active as you can and continue planning your celebrations for Day 29.

MENU

Breakfast
▨ 1 yellow Portion Pot® (30g) All-Bran served with milk from allowance and 1 tsp sugar, plus 1 boiled egg ☑

Mid-morning power snack
▨ ½ grapefruit sprinkled with 1 tsp sugar ☑

Lunch
▨ Stir-Fried Chicken: Stir-fry 100g chopped chicken breast (no skin) in a preheated non-stick wok or pan without any added fat. Add some crushed garlic and, when the chicken has changed colour and is almost cooked through, add some chopped peppers, celery, red onion, mushrooms and mangetout, taking care not to overcook the veg. Just before serving, add some grated ginger, soy sauce and fresh coriander and heat through 🄿
OR
▨ 1 slice wholegrain bread, toasted, topped with 1 × 300g can Heinz BBQ baked beans and 1 dry-fried small egg ☑

Mid-afternoon power snack
▨ 1 yellow Portion Pot® (125ml) apple juice

Dinner
▨ 1 × 150g lean lamb steak (raw weight) or 2 Quorn Lamb Style Grills, grilled, served with 115g boiled new potatoes (with skins), plus 200g other vegetables of your choice and a little low-fat gravy and mint sauce ☑
OR

- Wine Braised Pork Slices (see recipe, p.252) served with 115g boiled new potatoes (with skins) and additional other vegetables of your choice

Dessert
- 1 The Skinny Cow Triple Chocolate Stick

Alcohol or high-fat treat
- 50ml measure of gin or vodka with a Slimline mixer
OR
- 1 × 25g bag Walkers Squares Cheese & Onion Flavour Potato Snack

TEN-MINUTE TONE-UP – ADVANCED

See www.rosemaryconley.tv/ailpDay27

AEROBIC CHALLENGE

Do a 40-minute workout at a class or do a fitness DVD or go for a 60-minute brisk walk. Don't forget to stretch at the end.

Exercise tip
Plan to do tomorrow's exercises first thing in the morning, then they're done and you'll be less likely to sabotage your eating if you've risen early to work out.

MOTIVATIONAL THOUGHT FOR THE DAY

Today try on a garment that was a really tight fit on Day 1 and realise how many inches you have lost. It's very illuminating and satisfying to see the tangible difference in the fit of an item of clothing that was uncomfortably tight a month ago and that is very comfortably loose now.

Then pick up your 'weight-loss' bag in which you have placed the equivalent of your weight lost over the last three weeks and feel how heavy it is. Can you believe that you were once carrying that excess baggage around with you everywhere you went? No wonder you were tired and uncomfortable! In two days' time you will be adding even more weight to the bag and I hope you will be really impressed with your progress.

Try to work really hard today as every extra calorie you spend through activity will help minimise your body weight on the morning of Day 29 and maximise your results. Keep moving, keep smiling and look forward to your celebratory meal on Day 29.

Day 28

This is the last day of the 14-Day 1400 plan and perhaps the toughest bit of this eating plan. From tomorrow, though, if your personal calorie allowance permits, you will be able to eat more while continuing to lose weight. By the end of today you will have completed a very significant personal challenge and you can be proud of your efforts. Moreover you will have got your weight loss campaign off to a stunning start. Of course, you may not have much more weight to lose and you may even be happy with where you have now arrived, weight-wise. If so, please keep up the low-fat way of eating combined with regular activity so that it forms part of your everyday lifestyle.

Today's exercise plan runs through many of the toning exercises at their most challenging level and they will demonstrate how strong your muscles have become in just four weeks. Having strong muscles gives us a better shape and it makes weight loss and weight maintenance easier. Log on to www.rosemaryconley.tv/ailpDay28 and we'll work out together.

MENU

Breakfast
■ Fruit Smoothie: Blend 150g peaches, strawberries, raspberries or blueberries with 100g Total 2% fat Greek Yoghurt and milk from allowance ☑

Mid-morning power snack
■ 1 blue Portion Pot® (14g) Special K (eat dry or with milk from allowance) ☑

Lunch
■ 1 × 400g can any lentil or bean soup (max. 250 kcal and 5% fat), plus 1 piece fresh fruit (excluding bananas) ☑
OR
■ 1 pack Rosemary Conley Solo Slim® Soup: choose from Tomato, Pea and Ham, Three Bean and Chorizo, Mushroom, Lentil or Minestrone (order from www.rosemaryconley.com), plus 1 slice wholegrain bread and 1 piece fresh fruit ☑

Mid-afternoon power snack
■ 1 small bowl of mixed salad tossed in fat-free dressing ☑

Dinner
■ Sweet and Sour Pork Chop: Grill 1 × 140g lean pork chop, all visible fat removed, and serve with 115g boiled new potatoes (with skins), 100g each carrots and broccoli, plus 1 yellow Portion Pot® (125ml) Uncle Ben's Sweet & Sour Light sauce
OR
■ Barbecued Garlic Chicken (see recipe, p.244) served with 100g boiled new potatoes (with skins) plus salad or vegetables

Dessert
■ 1 meringue basket filled with 1 tsp 0% fat Greek yogurt and topped with 1 slice pineapple ☑

Alcohol or high-fat treat
■ 1 yellow Portion Pot® (125ml) glass champagne
OR
■ 1 × 20g fun-size bag M & Ms

TEN-MINUTE TONE-UP – ADVANCED

See www.rosemaryconley.tv/ailpDay28

AEROBIC CHALLENGE

Walk up and down stairs 5 times consecutively, twice throughout the day, plus take a 40-minute power walk or jog, or work out to a fitness DVD. Really go for it!

Exercise tip
Taking regular exercise will help to lower your cholesterol and blood pressure levels as well as burn extra calories and tone your muscles, so the benefits of continuing to exercise even after you have achieved your goal weight are enormous.

MOTIVATIONAL THOUGHT FOR THE DAY

Over the last four weeks you will have burned a lot of body fat through eating healthily and doing aerobic exercise. Your heart and lungs will have become fitter and more efficient and your skin will be looking much clearer.

The toning exercises that you have done almost every day will have strengthened your muscles considerably and caused them to become tighter and more efficient. If muscles are not worked, they will become smaller through wastage – and that's the last thing you need when you are trying to lose weight.

We need strong muscles for several reasons. Our muscles help us to move about, bend, carry things and complete all manner of functions in our everyday lives and if we don't keep our muscles strong, we will become weaker and less mobile. As muscle is energy-hungry tissue, so strong muscles also give us a higher metabolic rate, which helps us to burn extra calories every day even when we are not exercising.

Remember also that muscles are our 'fat-burning machines'. When we do aerobic activity, the extra oxygen we breathe in enters our bloodstream via our arteries and flows around our body and into our muscles. Then the mitochondria ('little engines') in our muscles spring into action and, with the aid of the oxygen, burn body fat to make fuel for energy. So, be assured, exercise is the key to weight loss and weight maintenance.

Do as much aerobic activity today as you can. The scales and the tape measure will show the benefits to your figure tomorrow if you do.

7 Phase 3: Your personal inch loss plan

Congratulations! You've done it! Four weeks of serious dieting and a major exercise programme completed. Now life gets a little easier as you move on to this third phase. You must be delighted with what you have achieved – lots of inches have disappeared from your body and no doubt a considerable amount of weight too.

Day 29

In the morning, after you have visited the bathroom, head for those scales. The results at the end of the fourth week on a diet are unpredictable. People lose weight at different rates and of course much depends on how accurate you have been in measuring your food portions, how much exercise you have done and how much you weighed in the first place.

Whatever you have lost – whether a big drop or just a few pounds – it is a significant milestone and you should be delighted. I really hope you are.

Now measure yourself with your tape measure or Magic Measure® and take a good look at how many inches you have lost from the different areas of your body. Get out your measuring belt and see where it fits around your waist. Record your results on your chart or in your journal.

Next, find something of equivalent weight to this week's loss to place in your 'weight-loss' bag, then lift it up. Savour the moment as you realise the superb results of your hard work and determination.

If possible, at some point today, take a photograph of yourself or get someone else to do it. Compare it with your original 'before' photograph that you took before you started the diet. The difference you can see should be very encouraging. From now on, take a photograph every month as you continue on the diet.

Working out your calorie allowance
To calculate your new personalised calorie allowance, turn to pages 378–9. Look at the column appropriate to your gender and age and then find your today's weight, or the nearest weight to it, on the table. This figure is your BMR (basal metabolic rate) calculation, which is the number of calories your body would burn if you stayed in bed all day and did nothing.

By eating this number of calories you will be meeting your basic metabolic needs and the bulk of those calories need to be taken in the form of proper, nutritious food – rather than alcohol, high-fat snacks or sugar. Your body will effectively then draw down your body fat to burn as extra fuel to make up the shortfall of calories you will be spending as you move about during the day and hopefully doing some exercise too.

As you lose each further half stone, you should adjust your calories accordingly. Sorry – but the slimmer you become, the fewer calories you have to eat if you want to keep losing weight at the same rate. An alternative would be to keep increasing your calorie output by doing extra exercise on top of what you are already doing.

Continue to exercise regularly. You can repeat the last two weeks of the 28-day exercise programme if you wish.

Alternatively, you can work out to my Real Results DVD, which includes a 20-minute aerobic workout and four different toning sections. Use this regularly and you will stay fit and strong. Choose any other activity you enjoy. As long as you combine some aerobic work with toning and strength exercises you will keep progressing and enjoying the benefits.

How to design your own plan

You can select any breakfast, lunch and dinner from the suggestions on the following pages. You will find more calorie-counted recipes on www.rosemaryconley.com and on our online TV channel www.rosemaryconley.tv where chef Dean Simpole-Clarke demonstrates how to prepare all the recipes in this book plus hundreds of additional low-fat recipes that will fit in with this diet.

For a diet to work it must offer foods that you enjoy. As long as the calories are counted and each meal is low in fat, you cannot go wrong. This diet has to be the most versatile ever. If there's a meal you don't like, you don't have to eat it, ever!

Always drink plenty of water and be sure to consume 450ml (¾ pint) skimmed or semi-skimmed milk every day to ensure you get sufficient calcium. Keep taking a multivitamin supplement just to be super-sure that you have all the necessary micronutrients for good health. If you eat similar foods all the time, because you like them, you could be missing out on some important vitamins and minerals.

If you have extra calories available, over and above the 1200 calories used within the basic diet, you can use these for an alcoholic drink, a low-fat dessert or treat and, remember, you can use 100 calories a day for a high-fat treat of your choice.

Don't exceed your daily calorie allowance unless you have saved up any calories during the week. It can be useful to have calories available for a party or special night out with friends, but if you abuse your treats allowance you will stop losing weight and you may find yourself falling back into old, high-fat, habits. It's just not worth it.

8 The 28-day plan diet menus

BREAKFASTS

Cereal breakfasts

▪ 1 green Portion Pot® (50g) Special K cereal plus milk from allowance and 1 tsp sugar ☑

▪ 1 yellow Portion Pot® (30g) fruit and fibre cereal served with milk from allowance and topped with 1 red Portion Pot® (115g) fresh raspberries or 1 tsp sugar ☑

▪ 1 red Portion Pot® (50g) fruit and fibre cereal (or any bran cereal), served with milk from allowance and 10 seedless grapes ☑

▪ 1 Weetabix or Shredded Wheat served with milk from allowance plus 1 tsp sugar and 1 thinly sliced medium banana ☑

▪ 2 Weetabix served with milk from allowance and 2 tsps sugar or 1 mini banana ☑

▪ 1 yellow Portion Pot® (14 Minis) Weetabix Fruit 'n' Nut Minis, plus 1 medium banana, sliced, served with milk from allowance ☑

▪ 1 yellow Portion Pot® (30g) All-Bran served with milk from allowance and 1 tsp sugar, plus 1 boiled egg ☑

▪ 1 red Portion Pot® (30g) Sugar Puffs mixed with 115g canned peaches in natural juice ☑

▪ Mix 100g 0% fat Greek yogurt with 1 blue Portion Pot® (40g) muesli and a little semi-skimmed milk from allowance to moisten. Add a little Silver Spoon Half Spoon to sweeten to taste. Leave to soak overnight in the refrigerator for best results. Serve chilled ☑

▦ 1 blue Portion Pot® (35g) uncooked porridge oats, cooked in water with 10 sultanas and served with milk from allowance ☑

Fruit breakfasts

▦ 1 Müllerlight yogurt, any flavour (max. 150 kcal), plus 1 small banana ☑

▦ 2 large bananas ☑

▦ Frozen Berry Smoothie (see recipe, p.272) ☑

▦ Fruit Smoothie: blend 150g fresh fruit (peaches, strawberries, raspberries or blueberries) with 100g Total 2% fat Greek Yoghurt and milk from allowance ☑

▦ 1 small banana, sliced, mixed with 115g sliced strawberries and 1 × 100g pot low-fat yogurt, any flavour (max. 100 kcal and 5% fat) ☑

▦ 200g fresh fruit salad topped with 100g Total 2% fat Greek Yoghurt and 6 sultanas ☑

▦ 100g Total 2% fat Greek Yoghurt mixed with 140g fresh fruit, sweetened to taste with a little Silver Spoon Half Spoon ☑

Quick and easy breakfasts

▦ 1 yellow Portion Pot® (125ml) fresh orange juice, plus 1 slice wholegrain bread spread with 2 tsps marmalade, jam or honey ☑

▦ ½ fresh grapefruit plus 2 boiled medium-sized eggs ☑ P

▦ ½ bagel (or 1 whole mini bagel) toasted, spread with 1 tsp fruit preserve, jam, honey or marmalade, then topped with 50g Total 2% fat Greek Yoghurt ☑

▦ 200g Total 2% fat Greek Yoghurt mixed with 1 tsp runny honey ☑

▦ 4 prunes, soaked overnight in 1 blue Portion Pot® (80g) low-fat natural yogurt, mixed with 1 tsp porridge oats ☑

Cooked breakfasts

■ 2 well-grilled back bacon rashers or 2 Quorn sausages, grilled, served with 1 dry-fried medium-sized egg, 3 tomatoes, halved and grilled, and 5 grilled mushrooms ☑P

■ 2 low-fat (max. 5% fat) beef, pork or Quorn sausages, grilled, served with 1 yellow Portion Pot® (115g) baked beans and 50g grilled mushrooms ☑P

■ 2 Quorn sausages, grilled, served with 1 dry-fried medium-sized egg and 1 × 200g can tomatoes, boiled until reduced ☑P

■ 2 Quorn sausages, grilled, served with 1 × 400g can tomatoes boiled until reduced, plus 50g grilled mushrooms ☑P

■ 1 Quorn Bacon Style Rasher, grilled, served with 1 yellow Portion Pot® (115g) baked beans plus 1 tomato, halved and grilled, and 50g grilled mushrooms ☑P

■ Tomatoes and Mushrooms on Toast: Boil 1 × 400g can chopped tomatoes well to reduce to a thick consistency and season well with freshly ground black pepper. Spoon onto 1 toasted large slice wholegrain bread and serve with 10 grilled mushrooms ☑

■ ½ fresh grapefruit plus 1 poached medium-sized egg served on 1 toasted small slice wholegrain bread spread with Marmite ☑

■ 2 eggs scrambled with milk from allowance and served with 100g grilled tomatoes and unlimited grilled mushrooms ☑P

■ 2-egg omelette made using milk from allowance, dry-fried and filled with chopped mushrooms, sliced cherry tomatoes and freshly ground black pepper ☑

■ 2 turkey rashers and 1 low-fat beef or pork sausage (max. 5% fat), grilled or dry-fried, served with 1 × 200g can tomatoes boiled until reduced and 100g grilled mushrooms P

■ 4 turkey rashers, grilled, served with 100g grilled, sliced mushrooms and 2 large tomatoes, grilled ☑P

■ 4 turkey rashers, grilled, served with 1 dry-fried medium-sized egg, 1 × 200g can plum tomatoes, boiled until reduced, and 5 grilled mushrooms **P**

■ 2 turkey rashers, grilled, served with 1 yellow Portion Pot® (115g) baked beans and 1 dry-fried medium-sized egg **P**

■ 1 slice wholegrain bread, toasted, topped with 1 yellow Portion Pot® (115g) baked beans ✔

■ 1 slice wholegrain bread, soaked in 1 beaten egg and milk from allowance, fried in a little spray oil and topped with 1 tsp maple syrup ✔

■ 1 small slice multigrain bread, toasted, served with 1 egg, scrambled, boiled or dry-fried; plus ½ pink grapefruit ✔

■ 1 slice wholegrain bread, toasted, spread with savoury sauce (e.g. tomato ketchup, brown sauce or fruity sauce), then topped with 2 grilled turkey rashers plus 3 grilled tomatoes

■ 1 slice wholegrain bread, toasted, topped with 1 scrambled egg and 2 grilled tomatoes ✔

■ 1 blue Portion Pot® (35g) uncooked porridge oats, cooked in water with 10 sultanas and served with milk from allowance ✔

LUNCHES

Sandwich lunches

■ Any pre-packed sandwich of your choice (max. 300 kcal and 5% fat) ✔

■ Spread 2 slices wholegrain bread with horseradish sauce or Hellmann's Extra Light Mayonnaise and make into a jumbo sandwich with 30g wafer thin beef, chicken or ham and salad vegetables

■ Cheese and Marmite Sandwich: Spread 2 slices wholegrain bread with Marmite and fill with 40g low-fat cottage cheese ✔

■ 1 medium slice wholegrain bread, toasted, topped with 1 × 125g can sardines or mackerel fillets, plus a small salad

■ BLT Sandwich: Toast 2 slices wholegrain bread, then spread 1 slice with 1 tsp Hellmann's Extra Light Mayonnaise and the other with tomato ketchup and fill with 25g lean grilled bacon, 1 slice wafer thin chicken, lettuce leaves and sliced tomatoes

■ Spread 2 slices wholegrain bread with HP Fruity Sauce (or similar) and make into a sandwich with 3 grilled turkey rashers, then toast in a sandwich toaster or double-sided electric grill

Rolls, bagels and baguettes

■ 1 small wholegrain roll spread with 1 tsp horseradish sauce and topped with 50g wafer thin beef and sliced tomatoes, plus a small salad tossed in fat-free dressing

■ 1 bagel cut in half, spread with 50g Philadelphia Extra Light soft cheese then topped with 50g smoked salmon and freshly ground black pepper or chopped fresh dill

■ 1 small granary baguette spread with 1 tsp horseradish sauce mixed with a little low-fat Greek yogurt and filled with 100g diced cooked beetroot, 50g smoked trout fillets plus rocket leaves and watercress

■ 1 × 40g granary baguette spread with 20g Philadelphia Extra Light soft cheese then topped with 25g wafer thin ham or Quorn Deli Ham Style, 1 sliced tomato and mustard to taste, plus a small side salad ☑

■ BLT Bruschetta: Cut 1 × 30g granary or wholegrain baguette in half and toast lightly, then spread with 2 tsps Hellmann's Extra Light Mayonnaise. Top with lettuce, sliced tomato and 2 × 15g extra lean grilled back bacon rashers

Pitta bread and wraps

■ 1 × 50g wholemeal pitta bread filled with 50g low-fat houmous and chopped mixed salad sprinkled with low-fat dressing of your choice ☑

■ 1 pitta bread, split open, then spread with low-fat Marie Rose dressing or very low-fat mayonnaise and filled with shredded lettuce, cherry tomatoes and 100g cooked prawns

■ Brunch Pitta (see recipe, p.254)

■ Prawn Wrap: Spread 1 tortilla wrap with 1 tsp Thai sweet chilli dipping sauce, then fill with 50g cooked prawns, chopped salad leaves, peppers, cucumber, celery and cherry tomatoes and wrap into a parcel before cutting in half horizontally to make 2 wraps

■ 1 tortilla wrap spread with 1 tsp Thai sweet chilli dipping sauce, then filled with 50g cooked prawns, chopped salad leaves, peppers, cucumber, celery and cherry tomatoes and wrapped into a parcel before cutting in half horizontally to make 2 wraps

■ Greek Salad Wrap (see recipe, p266) ☑

Salad lunches

■ 100g cooked chicken breast (no skin), sliced, served with a large mixed salad and 1 tbsp Hellmann's Extra Light Mayonnaise **P**

■ Mixed Bean Salad: Mix together 100g drained, canned chickpeas, 100g red kidney beans and 25g sweetcorn kernels. Add 2 sliced spring onions, 3 halved cherry tomatoes, unlimited chopped celery, peppers and cucumber, and mix well. Stir in some chopped fresh coriander and basil and toss in balsamic vinegar or fat-free dressing of your choice and add freshly ground black pepper to taste ☑

■ 2 hard-boiled eggs served with salad of chopped vegetables and salad leaves, tossed in low-fat dressing of your choice. Plus 1 kiwi fruit and 1 small pear ☑ **P**

■ 100g cooked prawns served with a large mixed salad and 1 tbsp low-fat thousand island dressing. Plus 1 Danone Shape Lasting Satisfaction or Weight Watchers yogurt, any flavour

■ Large salad of grated carrots, beansprouts, chopped peppers, celery, tomatoes, cucumber and red onion, served with 1 blue Portion Pot® (100g) low-fat cottage cheese, plus 1 tbsp Hellmann's Extra Light Mayonnaise. Plus 1 low-fat yogurt (max. 100 kcal and 5% fat) ☑

■ Salad Bowl with Prawns, Chicken or Ham: Place a large selection of shredded salad leaves and fresh herbs such as coriander and basil in a serving dish. Add layers of chopped peppers, onion, celery, mushrooms, cucumber and cherry tomatoes and top with chopped fresh fruits such as pineapple, papaya, mango, kiwi. Add 50g cooked prawns or chicken or shredded ham, then pour some low-fat Marie Rose sauce or other low-fat dressing over the salad and sprinkle with chopped chives ℗

■ Large mixed salad plus 1 smoked mackerel fillet or 1 × 125g can sardines or salmon (not in oil), served with 2 tsps Hellmann's Extra Light Mayonnaise or other low-fat dressing of your choice. Plus 1 pear or orange ℗

Quick and easy lunches
■ 1 egg, scrambled, then mixed with 25g Rosemary Conley low-fat Mature Cheese and served on 1 toasted small slice multigrain bread with 1 sliced tomato

■ ½ × 410g can Stagg Vegetable Garden Vegetable Chilli and 1 small wholegrain roll plus a small salad tossed in fat-free dressing ☑

■ 1 slice wholegrain bread, toasted, topped with 1 × 300g can Heinz BBQ baked beans and 1 dry-fried small egg ☑

■ 200g Total 2% fat Greek Yoghurt mixed with 1 tsp runny honey and 1 red Portion Pot® (115g) raspberries or chopped strawberries or 1 yellow Portion Pot® (70g) blueberries, topped with 1 tsp muesli ☑℗

■ 1 yellow Portion Pot® (115g) baked beans served on 2 toasted slices multigrain bread ✓

Cooked lunches

■ 1 × 140g tuna steak, grilled, served with 100g cooked peas and 50g sweetcorn plus a small salad. Plus 100g Total 2 % fat Greek Yoghurt mixed with 1 red Portion Pot® (115g) raspberries

■ 2-egg omelette made using milk from allowance and lots of freshly ground black pepper, filled with chopped peppers, red onion, mushrooms and 25g grated low-fat cheese (max. 5 % fat, e.g. Rosemary Conley low-fat Mature Cheese) ✓ P

■ Spanish omelette: In a non-stick frying pan or omelette pan, cook 2 beaten eggs with chopped peppers and red onion and 1 sliced, small cooked new potato. Serve with a small mixed salad tossed in fat-free dressing ✓

■ 2 well-grilled back bacon rashers, served with 1 dry-fried medium-sized egg, 1 × 400g can plum tomatoes boiled and reduced and 100g grilled or boiled mushrooms

■ Chicken or Quorn Stir-Fry: Dry-fry 100g sliced chicken breast (no skin) or Quorn fillets in a non-stick pan, then add a selection of chopped vegetables (e.g. peppers, onions, carrots, courgettes, celery, beansprouts), plus soy sauce to taste and 2 tsps sweet chilli sauce, taking care not to overcook the vegetables. Plus 1 low-fat yogurt (max. 100 kcal and 5 % fat) ✓ P

■ Turkey and Mango Samosas (see recipe, p.247) served with unlimited fresh vegetables or salad

■ Gammon and Liver Kebabs: Cut 1 × 100g gammon steak (all visible fat removed) and 125g lamb's liver into bite-sized pieces and thread alternately on to wooden skewers. Cook under a hot conventional grill for 3–4 minutes each side or in a health grill for 2 minutes. Serve with grilled tomatoes and mixed salad leaves P

■ Stir-Fried Chicken: Stir-fry 100g chopped chicken breast (no skin) in a preheated non-stick wok or pan without any added fat. Add some crushed garlic and, when the chicken has changed colour and is almost cooked through, add some chopped peppers, celery, red onion, mushrooms and mangetout, taking care not to overcook the vegetables. Just before serving, add some grated ginger, soy sauce and fresh coriander and heat through **P**

■ 2 low-fat beef or pork sausages (max. 5% fat) or 2 Quorn sausages, grilled, served with 1 yellow Portion Pot® (115g) baked beans, 1 dry-fried small egg, 1 small can tomatoes boiled well to reduce, plus unlimited grilled or boiled mushrooms ☑**P**

■ 1 × 175g oven-baked sweet potato topped with either 75g tuna or low-fat cottage cheese, mixed with 1 tbsp sweetcorn and 1 tbsp Hellmann's Extra Light Mayonnaise, served with a small salad tossed in fat-free dressing of your choice ☑

■ 1 × 175g oven-baked sweet potato topped with 75g baked beans, served with a side salad tossed in fat-free dressing of your choice ☑

Pasta, rice and noodle lunches

■ Chicken Pasta: Cook 1 yellow Portion Pot® (45g dry weight) pasta shapes, then mix with 50g cooked, chopped chicken breast (no skin). Add some chopped salad vegetables (onions, peppers, cucumber, tomatoes), mix in 4 tbsps Hellmann's Extra Light Mayonnaise and serve with a small mixed salad

■ Tuna or Chicken Pasta Salad: 1 red Portion Pot® (110g cooked weight) pasta shapes mixed with either 50g drained canned tuna (in brine) or 30g chopped cooked chicken breast, plus unlimited chopped peppers, red onion, cucumber, tomato and celery and 2 tsps Hellmann's Extra Light Mayonnaise or low-fat thousand island dressing

■ Pasta with Tomato and Basil Sauce: Boil 1 yellow Portion Pot® (45g uncooked weight) pasta shapes in water with a vegetable stock cube, then drain and mix with ½ × 340g jar (170g) tomato and basil pasta sauce ☑

■ Smoked Salmon Pasta Salad: Toss 1 yellow Portion Pot® (45g uncooked weight) or 1 red Portion Pot® (110g cooked weight) boiled pasta shapes with 50g smoked salmon strips and 1 yellow Portion Pot® (135g) low-fat fromage frais and chopped fresh dill, and serve with a green salad

■ Garlic Mushroom Pasta (see recipe, p.260) ☑

■ Singapore Noodles with Prawns (see recipe, p.257) plus a crisp salad ☑

■ Stir-Fried Rice Noodles (see recipe, p.264) served with salad ☑

■ 75g cooked egg noodles tossed with unlimited beansprouts, spring onions, chopped peppers, fresh coriander and 75g flaked cooked salmon, served with soy sauce

■ Chicken and Rice Salad: 80g (cooked weight) boiled basmati rice mixed with 60g cooked chopped chicken breast (no skin), chopped peppers, red onion, mushrooms, celery and 1 tbsp sweetcorn kernels. Season with freshly ground black pepper and soy sauce or fat-free dressing of your choice

■ Bombay Rice (see recipe, p.263) served with salad ☑

Soup lunches

■ 1 × 400g can any soup (max. 150 kcal and 5% fat). Plus 1 Müllerlight yogurt, any flavour (max. 150 kcal)

■ 1 can any lentil or bean soup (max. 200 kcal and 5% fat); followed by 2 pieces fresh fruit (excluding bananas) ☑

■ 1 Batchelors Cup a Soup. Plus 1 Müllerlight yogurt (max. 150 kcal) and 1 kiwi fruit

■ Chicken Noodle Soup (see recipe, p.242) served with 1 small wholegrain pitta bread, toasted

■ Homemade Vegetable Soup (makes enough for approx. 6 servings): Bring 2 litres of water to the boil in a large pan, then add 2 vegetable stock cubes and 400g peeled and trimmed vegetables (e.g. carrots, parsnips, onion, cabbage) or leftover vegetables and boil until cooked. Remove from the heat, add some chopped coriander and black pepper and leave to cool a little. Pour the soup in small batches into a food processor and blend for a few seconds, then transfer to a storage container or jug and allow to cool before storing or freezing. Reheat as required, allowing 300ml per serving and accompany with a slice of toasted wholegrain bread ☑

■ Broccoli and Leek Soup (see recipe, p.240) served with a small granary roll ☑

■ Chicken, Mushroom and Lemon Soup (see recipe, p.241) served with a small wholegrain roll (max. 150 kcal). Plus 1 pear or orange

■ 1 pack Rosemary Conley Solo Slim® Soup: choose from flavours including Tomato, Pea and Ham, Three Bean and Chorizo, Mushroom, Lentil or Minestrone (order from www.rosemaryconley.com), plus 1 slice wholegrain bread and 1 piece fresh fruit. See p.318 for more Rosemary Conley Solo Slim® lunch options

DINNERS

Chicken and turkey dinners

■ Chinese Chicken Kebabs (see recipe, p.243) served with 1 blue Portion Pot® (55g uncooked weight) or 1 red Portion Pot® (144g cooked weight) basmati rice per person

■ Mixed Grill: 4 turkey rashers and 1 low-fat sausage, grilled, served with 1 dry-fried egg, 1 yellow Portion Pot® (115g) baked beans, unlimited grilled mushrooms plus 1 × 400g can tomatoes boiled well to reduce 🅿

■ Chicken with Couscous: Season 1 × 120g skinless chicken breast with a little salt and plenty of freshly ground black pepper, then grill, steam or microwave. Serve with 1 blue Portion Pot® (50g uncooked weight) steamed couscous, plus unlimited salad or vegetables and 2 tsps Thai sweet chilli dipping sauce or mango chutney

■ 150g roast chicken breast (no skin) served with 100g dry-roast sweet potatoes plus 200g other vegetables of your choice (e.g. carrots, broccoli, cauliflower) and low-fat gravy

■ Quick and Easy Chicken Curry: Dry-fry 1 × 115g chopped chicken breast (no skin) in a preheated non-stick pan with ½ chopped onion and 1 crushed garlic clove. Sprinkle 1 tsp curry powder over and 'cook out' for 1 minute, then add 1 small chopped chilli, ½ chopped green pepper, 25g button mushrooms (optional) and 1 × 400g can chopped tomatoes, and simmer for 5 minutes to reduce. Serve with 1 blue Portion Pot® (55g uncooked weight) or 1 red Portion Pot® (144g cooked weight) basmati rice

■ Chicken in Mushroom Sauce: Dry-fry 100g chopped chicken breast (no skin) with ½ chopped onion and 6 button mushrooms. When the chicken is almost cooked, add 100g (⅓ can) Batchelors Low Fat Condensed Mushroom Soup, plus milk from allowance if needed to make a creamy sauce. Simmer until the chicken is completely cooked. Serve with 1 yellow Portion Pot® (100g) mashed sweet potato, plus other vegetables of your choice

■ Barbecued Garlic Chicken (see recipe, p.244) served with 100g boiled new potatoes (with skins) plus salad or vegetables

■ Spicy Chicken Pasta: Dry-fry 110g chopped chicken breast (no skin) and ½ chopped onion in a non-stick wok and season with freshly ground black pepper. Add 1 crushed garlic clove, 1 sliced green pepper, 1 × 400g can chopped tomatoes, ½ small chopped chilli and a dash of Worcestershire sauce and allow to simmer for 5 minutes. Serve with 1 yellow Portion Pot® (45g uncooked weight) or 1 red Portion Pot® (110g cooked weight) pasta shapes

■ Stir-Fry Chicken with Ginger: Chop 100g chicken breast (no skin) into bite-sized pieces and dry-fry in a non-stick pan with ½ crushed garlic clove. When the chicken has changed colour and is almost cooked through, add 1 chopped red or green pepper, 1 chopped celery stick, ½ chopped red onion, 25g mushrooms and 50g mangetout and dry-fry quickly but do not overcook. Just before serving add 1 tsp grated fresh ginger, soy sauce to taste and 1 tsp grated fresh coriander and heat through **P**

■ Southern Fried Turkey (see recipe, p.246) served hot with unlimited vegetables (excluding potatoes) or salad **P**

■ Chicken Shaslik (see recipe, p.245) served with 1 blue Portion Pot® (55g uncooked weight) or 1 red Portion Pot® (144g cooked weight) basmati rice per person

Beef dinners
■ 100g lean roast beef, thinly sliced, served with 100g dry-roasted potatoes and 200g other vegetables of your choice (excluding potatoes), plus low-fat gravy and 1 tsp horseradish sauce

■ Beef Kebabs: Cut 150g rump steak into bite-sized pieces and thread on to wooden skewers with 8 chestnut mushrooms, then baste with 50g tomato passata and 1 tsp balti curry paste. Cook the kebabs for 5–6 minutes in a health grill or 10 minutes under a conventional grill. Check the centre of meat is cooked and, when ready to serve, sprinkle with ½ tbsp chopped fresh coriander and serve with fresh green vegetables or salad **P**

■ 175g lean beef fillet or rump steak, grilled, served with a large salad plus 1 tbsp Hellmann's Extra Light Mayonnaise **P**

■ Beef Fajitas: Dry-fry 120g sliced lean beef with ½ each sliced red and green pepper and ½ chopped red onion, then mix in 2 tsps fajita spice mix. Fill a low-fat tortilla wrap with the mixture and serve with 1 blue Portion Pot® (75g) tomato salsa and a large mixed salad tossed in oil-free dressing

■ Steak in Mushroom Sauce: Dry-fry 2 thin beef steaks (250g total) quickly on both sides. Remove from the pan and keep warm. Add 100g chestnut mushrooms to the pan and cook for 1 minute before adding 1 tsp Knorr Touch of Taste beef stock and 75ml water. Bring the sauce to the boil and reduce by half. Remove from the heat and stir in ½ tbsp 3 % fat yogurt. Transfer the steaks to a serving plate and top with the mushroom sauce. Serve with green vegetables or salad **P**

■ Cheesy Cottage Pie (see recipe, p.249)

■ Pasta Bolognese: Dry-fry 100g lean minced beef in a non-stick pan, seasoning well with black pepper. Drain off the fat, add ½ chopped onion, 1 crushed garlic clove and ½ chopped red pepper and dry-fry until soft. Stir in ¼ jar Dolmio Bolognese Original Light Pasta Sauce and 1 × 200g can chopped tomatoes and simmer for 10 minutes. Serve with 1 yellow Portion Pot® (45g uncooked weight) pasta shapes, boiled with a vegetable stock cube

■ Baked Liver and Onions: Place 150g calves' liver in an ovenproof dish with 1 sliced onion. Cover with foil and cook in a moderate oven (180C, 350F, Gas Mark 4) for 15–20 minutes until lightly cooked. Make some low-fat gravy with gravy powder and add to the liver and onion. Serve with 1 yellow Portion Pot® (100g) mashed potato and other vegetables of your choice

Pork dinners

■ Ham, Leek and Sweet Potato Pie (see recipe, p.253) served with unlimited vegetables (excluding potatoes) or salad

■ Ham and Cheese Omelette: Beat 3 eggs with milk from allowance and cook in a non-stick pan. Add 25g grated Rosemary Conley low-fat Mature Cheese and 25g shredded ham. Serve with a large salad tossed in fat-free dressing **P**

■ 1 × 150g (raw weight) lean pork steak (all visible fat removed), grilled, served with 115g boiled new potatoes (with skins), 200g other vegetables of your choice, plus low-fat gravy and 1 tbsp apple sauce

■ Spicy Pork Steak: Mix together 1 tsp ground cumin, 1 tsp ground ginger and 1 tsp smoked paprika on a plate, then press 300g lean pork steak into the spices and season with salt and pepper. Cook the steak in a health grill for 8–10 minutes or under a conventional grill for 8–10 minutes each side. Serve hot with a mixed salad or vegetables of your choice **P**

■ Wine Braised Pork Slices (see recipe, p.252) served with 115g boiled new potatoes (with skins) and additional other vegetables of your choice

■ Sweet and Sour Pork Chop: Grill 1 × 140g lean pork chop, all visible fat removed, and serve with 115g boiled new potatoes (with skins), 100g each carrots and broccoli, plus 1 yellow Portion Pot® (125ml) Uncle Ben's Sweet & Sour Light sauce

■ 1 × 115g lean pork steak (all visible fat removed), grilled, served with 1 yellow Portion Pot® (100g) mashed sweet potato, plus unlimited other vegetables and low-fat gravy

■ 3 low-fat pork sausages, grilled, served with 1 yellow Portion Pot® (100g) mashed, sweet potatoes plus unlimited vegetables and low-fat gravy

Lamb dinners

■ 1 × 150g lean lamb steak (raw weight), grilled, served with 115g boiled new potatoes (with skins), plus 200g other vegetables of your choice and a little low-fat gravy and mint sauce

■ Lamb and Mushroom Goulash (see recipe, p.251) served with green vegetables

■ Lamb Stir-Fry: Cut 150g lean lamb steak into strips and dry-fry with ½ chopped onion and ½ crushed garlic clove in a non-stick pan over a high heat for 1–2 minutes. Add 1 tsp mint sauce, 75g stir-fry vegetables and ½ tbsp soy sauce and toss well before cooking for 7–8 minutes. Serve on a bed of lightly cooked beansprouts **P**

■ Lamb Medallions with Blackcurrant Sauce (see recipe, p.248) served with 100g boiled new potatoes (with skins) and unlimited vegetables

Fish and seafood dinners

■ 150g cod fillet, microwaved or steamed, and 50g cooked prawns, served with ½ × 300g pack (150g) Schwartz for Fish low-fat Chunky Tomato, Olive and Rosemary Sauce, plus unlimited carrots and broccoli or courgettes and 1 yellow Portion Pot® (70g) peas **P**

■ 150g tuna steak, grilled, served with 1 blue Portion Pot® (50g uncooked weight) couscous (any flavour, e.g. see Ainsley Harriott range) plus 1 blue Portion Pot® (75g) tomato salsa and a large salad

■ Oven-Baked Salmon: Place 1 × 110g salmon steak in an ovenproof dish, top with 1 tsp Thai sweet chilli dipping sauce and the juice of ½ lime. Bake in a preheated oven at 200C, 400F, Gas Mark 6 for 8–10 minutes, or until cooked. Serve with 100g boiled new potatoes (with skins) and unlimited green vegetables

■ 1 × 115g (raw weight) salmon steak, steamed or microwaved, served with 80g boiled new potatoes (with skins), plus 1 yellow Portion Pot® (70g) frozen or canned peas, 100g steamed broccoli or asparagus and 1 tbsp Hellmann's Extra Light Mayonnaise

■ Fish Pie: Place 50g each of fresh salmon, cod and shelled uncooked prawns in a small ovenproof dish and cover with ⅓ can Batchelors Low Fat Condensed Mushroom Soup, top with mashed potato (made by boiling 115g old potatoes then mashing with milk from allowance and seasoning well). Place in the oven and bake at 200C, 400F, Gas Mark 6 for 30 minutes or until the potato is browned on top. Serve with unlimited carrots and broccoli **P**

■ Chilli Prawn Stir-Fry with Peppers and Mushrooms: Dry-fry 150g fresh prawns in a non-stick wok. When they have changed colour, add ½ each chopped red and green pepper, 5 button mushrooms, 1 chopped celery stick, ½ chopped red onion, 1 small courgette, chopped, and ½ pack of fresh (or 1 whole can) beansprouts. Do not overcook. Just before serving add 1 tbsp Thai sweet chilli dipping sauce and soy sauce to taste. Plus 1 low-fat yogurt or other low-fat dessert (max. 100 kcal and 5% fat) **P**

■ Prawn Saag (see recipe, p.256) served with 1 green Portion Pot® (170g) cooked egg noodles or 1 blue Portion Pot® (55g uncooked weight) or 1 red Portion Pot® (144g cooked weight) basmati rice per person. Plus 1 meringue nest topped with 1 tbsp 0% fat Greek yogurt and 2 sliced strawberries

■ Black Bean Prawns (see recipe, p.255) served with 1 blue Portion Pot® (55g uncooked weight) or 1 red Portion Pot® (144g cooked weight) basmati rice. Plus 1 Marks & Spencer meringue nest topped with 1 tsp 0% fat Greek yogurt and 1 tbsp raspberries

■ Chilli Prawn Stir-Fry with Asparagus: Dry-fry ½ chopped red onion and ½ crushed garlic clove in a non-stick pan until soft. Add 50g sliced asparagus and 100g uncooked, shelled prawns and continue cooking for 2–3 minutes. Pour in 1 × 75g pack chilli stir-fry sauce and stir well to coat the prawns and vegetables. Bring to the boil, then turn off the heat. Serve with salad and garnish with fresh chives

Vegetarian dinners

■ Quorn Bolognese: Dry-fry 100g Quorn mince in a non-stick pan, seasoning well with black pepper. Add ½ chopped onion, 1 crushed garlic clove and ½ chopped red pepper and dry-fry until soft. Stir in ¼ jar Dolmio Bolognese Original Light Pasta Sauce and 1 × 200g can chopped tomatoes and simmer for 10 minutes. Serve with 1 yellow Portion Pot® (45g uncooked weight) pasta shapes, boiled with a vegetable stock cube **P**

■ Pasta Ratatouille: In a saucepan, mix together 1 small can of tomatoes, 2 tsps tomato purée, ½ chopped red onion, ½ chopped red or green pepper, ½ chopped aubergine and ½ sliced courgette. Sprinkle with 1 tsp oregano and some chopped fresh basil and simmer for 15–20 minutes, adding a little vegetable stock if required. When the vegetables are tender, mix in 1 red Portion Pot® (110g cooked weight) boiled pasta shapes and heat through **✓**

■ Vegetable Chilli: Dry-fry 1 chopped onion in a preheated non-stick pan. Add 1 × 200g can mixed beans in chilli sauce and 1 × 200g can chopped tomatoes plus chopped vegetables (e.g. courgettes, mushrooms, carrots, peppers) and simmer for 15–20 minutes. Serve with 1 blue Portion Pot® (55g uncooked weight) or 1 red Portion Pot® (144g cooked weight) basmati rice **✓**

■ 2 Quorn Peppered Steaks, grilled, served with a large salad plus 1 tbsp Hellmann's Extra Light Mayonnaise **✓P**

■ 2 Quorn Lamb Style Grills, grilled, served with 115g boiled new potatoes (with skins), plus 200g other vegetables of your choice and a little low-fat gravy and mint sauce **✓**

■ 1 × 200g oven-baked sweet potato topped with 200g baked beans and served with a side salad tossed in low-fat dressing of your choice ☑

■ Cheesy Quorn Bake: Dry-fry 1 finely chopped red onion and 1 crushed garlic clove in a non-stick pan until soft, then stir in 100g Quorn mince and cook for a further 2 minutes. Add 200g chopped tomatoes, 250g tomato passata, ½–1 tsp vegetable stock powder, ½ tbsp chives and reduce to a gentle simmer. While the Quorn mixture is simmering, heat a non-stick griddle pan and cook 150g chopped courgettes on both sides until lightly browned, seasoning with black pepper. Layer the courgettes and Quorn mixture in an ovenproof dish. Pour 150g 2% fat Greek yogurt over the top and add 25g grated Rosemary Conley low-fat Mature Cheese and black pepper to taste. Bake in a preheated oven at 200C, 400F, Gas Mark 6 for 20 minutes until the cheese has melted and the dish is hot all the way through. Garnish with chopped chives ☑ P

■ Sweet and Sour Quorn: Dry-fry ½ × 350g pack Quorn Chicken Style Pieces (175g) with ½ chopped onion, ½ each chopped red and green pepper, 5 button mushrooms, halved, 1 chopped celery stick and 1 small chopped courgette. Add 1 yellow Portion Pot® (125ml) Uncle Ben's Sweet & Sour Light sauce and heat through before serving. Plus 1 low-fat yogurt or other dessert (max. 100 kcal and 5% fat) ☑ P

■ ½ pack any branded fresh filled pasta (max. 5% fat) served with ½ pot ready-made low-fat fresh tomato-based sauce (max. 400 kcal total for whole meal) ☑

■ 2 Quorn sausages, grilled, served with ½ pack readymade cauliflower cheese (max. 200 kcal and 5% fat) and green vegetables of your choice ☑

■ 3 Quorn sausages, grilled, served with 1 yellow Portion Pot® (100g) mashed sweet potatoes, plus unlimited other vegetables and a little low-fat gravy ☑

■ Quorn and Rice Bake (see recipe, p.262) served with unlimited vegetables (excluding potatoes) ☑

■ Chilli Quorn Stir-Fry with Asparagus: Dry-fry ½ chopped red onion and ½ crushed garlic clove in a non-stick pan until soft. Add 50g sliced asparagus and 100g Quorn pieces and continue cooking for 2–3 minutes. Pour in 1 × 75g pack chilli stir-fry sauce and stir well to coat the Quorn pieces and the vegetables. Bring to the boil, then turn off the heat. Serve with salad and garnish with fresh chives ☑ P

■ 1 low-fat veggie burger (max. 180 kcal and 5% fat, e.g. Grassington's Vegetable Quarter Pounder or Quorn Quarter Pounder) cooked as per instructions. Serve with 115g boiled new potatoes (with skins) and a large salad tossed in low-fat dressing ☑

■ Pasta with Tomato and Basil Sauce: Mix 1 red Portion Pot® (80g uncooked weight) or 1 green Portion Pot® (176g cooked weight) boiled pasta shapes with ½ jar (approx. 200g) ready-made tomato and basil pasta sauce and heat through. Serve with chopped fresh basil leaves and a sprinkling of Parmesan shavings, plus a large green salad tossed in fat-free dressing ☑

■ Roasted Pepper Pasta (see recipe, p.261) served with a large salad tossed in fat-free dressing ☑

■ Leek and Sage Meatballs with Pasta (see recipe, p.258)

■ Cauliflower Bhaji (see recipe, p.265) served with 1 blue Portion Pot® (55g uncooked weight) or 1 red Portion Pot® (144g cooked weight) basmati rice per person ☑

■ Any low-fat vegetarian ready meal (max. 400 kcal and 5% fat, including any accompaniments) ☑

Ready meals

▦ 1 × 400g pack Asda Good For You Chilli Beef & Mushrooms. Serve with green salad tossed in fat-free dressing

▦ 1 × 400g pack Asda Good For You Spicy Tomato Chicken. Plus 1 low-fat yogurt (max. 120 kcal and 5% fat)

▦ 1 × 400g pack Asda Good For You Chicken Chasseur. Serve with unlimited vegetables (excluding potatoes)

▦ 1 × 450g pack Asda Good For You Chicken Tikka Masala & Pilau Rice

▦ 1 × 400g pack Sainsbury's Be Good To Yourself Chicken Tikka Masala with Pilau Rice

▦ 1 × 400g pack Sainsbury's Be Good To Yourself Lasagne. Serve with green salad tossed in fat-free dressing

▦ 1 × 400g pack Sainsbury's Be Good To Yourself Chicken and Pasta Bake. Serve with green salad tossed in fat-free dressing

▦ 1 × 400g pack Asda Good For You Chicken & Broccoli. Serve with unlimited green vegetables

▦ 1 × 375g pack Morrisons Eat Smart Diet Chicken in Peppercorn Sauce with Sliced Roast Potatoes. Serve with unlimited green vegetables

▦ 1 × 375g pack Morrisons Chicken in Tomato and Basil Sauce. Serve with unlimited vegetables (excluding potatoes)

▦ 1 × 400g pack Morrisons Eat Smart Chicken Korma with Pilau Rice

▦ Marks & Spencer Count On Us Steak Yorkshires (1 pudding per person). Serve with 100g lean roast beef and unlimited green vegetables and low-fat gravy

▦ 1 × 400g pack Marks & Spencer Count On Us Cajun Chicken Fettucine. Serve with green salad tossed in fat-free dressing

▦ 1 × 400g pack Marks & Spencer Count On Us Braised Beef in Ale. Serve with green vegetables.

▦ 1 × 400g pack Marks & Spencer Count on Us King Prawn Masala. Serve with green salad tossed in fat-free dressing

■ 1 × 400g pack Waitrose Low Saturated Fat Chicken & Asparagus with Roast Potatoes

■ 1 × 395g pack Waitrose Low Saturated Fat Chicken Korma with Pilau Rice

■ Any meal from Rosemary Conley's Solo Slim® range (order from www.rosemaryconley.com; and see p.323 for more Rosemary Conley Solo Slim® dinner options):

☐ 1 × 300g pack Rosemary Conley Solo Slim® Beef Meatballs and Potato. Serve with unlimited vegetables (excluding potatoes)

☐ 1 × 300g pack Rosemary Conley Solo Slim® Lamb Hotpot. Plus 1 low-fat yogurt (max. 150 kcal and 5% fat)

☐ 1 × 300g pack Rosemary Conley Solo Slim® Chilli and Rice. Serve with 1 × 50g crusty wholegrain roll

☐ 1 × 300g pack Rosemary Conley Solo Slim® Spicy Vegetable and Lentil Dahl. Plus 1 low-fat yogurt (max. 150 kcal and 5% fat) ☑

POWER SNACKS

Fruit

■ 1 whole papaya, peeled and deseeded ☑

■ 100g cherries ☑

■ 75g fresh mango ☑

■ 12 seedless grapes ☑

■ 1 medium pear ☑

■ 100g fresh pineapple ☑

■ 1 × 200g slice melon (weighed without skin) ☑

■ 150g strawberries ☑

■ 1 small apple ☑

■ 2 kiwi fruit ☑

■ 2 dried apricots ☑

■ 20g sultanas ☑

- 1 kid's fun-size mini banana ☑
- 1 kiwi fruit plus 5 seedless grapes ☑
- 2 satsumas ☑
- 2 plums ☑
- ½ grapefruit sprinkled with 1 tsp sugar ☑
- 150g fresh fruit salad ☑
- 1 red Portion Pot® (115g) raspberries plus 50g strawberries ☑
- 1 yellow Portion Pot® (70g) blueberries plus 1 tsp low-fat natural yogurt ☑
- 1 yellow Portion Pot® (125ml) fresh orange or apple juice ☑
- 1 red Portion Pot® (115g) raspberries topped with 2 tsps low-fat yogurt (max. 5% fat) ☑
- 1 × 90g pack Tesco Fresh Apple and Grape Snack Pack ☑
- 100g any stewed fruit sweetened with low-cal sweetener ☑

Sweet
- 1 fat-free yogurt, any flavour (max. 50 kcal) ☑
- 1 Hartley's Low Calorie Jelly topped with 1 tbsp Total 2% Greek Yoghurt and 3 berries of your choice
- 1 blue Portion Pot® (14g) Special K (eat dry or with milk from allowance) ☑
- 1 Caxton Pink 'n' Whites wafer ☑

Savoury
- 1 rice cake spread with 20g Philadelphia Extra Light soft cheese and sliced cucumber ☑
- 5 mini low-fat bread sticks plus 1 tsp (25g) Total 0% fat Greek Yoghurt mixed with chopped chives ☑
- 1 Asda Good For You Chicken Noodle Cup Soup
- 10 sweet silverskin pickled onions plus 10 cherry tomatoes ☑
- 20g low-fat cheese (max. 5% fat) plus 5 cherry tomatoes ☑
- 1 Rakusen's cracker topped with 1 × 20g triangle Laughing Cow Extra Light soft cheese, plus 5 cherry tomatoes

- 1 Ryvita spread thinly with Philadelphia Extra Light soft cheese ☑
- 1 Ryvita, spread with Marmite and topped with 2 tsps low-fat cottage cheese ☑
- 1 blue Portion Pot® (75g) tomato salsa plus 1 carrot, 1 celery stick and 1 × 5cm piece cucumber sliced into crudités ☑
- 2 carrots, cut into sticks, served with 1 tbsp low-fat yogurt mixed with fresh chopped chives and finely chopped red onion ☑
- 10 cherry tomatoes, plus chunks of carrots, cucumber and green or red pepper ☑
- 1 small bowl of mixed salad tossed in fat-free dressing ☑

DESSERTS

All the following desserts are less than 5% fat.

Ice cream and iced desserts
- Strawberry and Rhubarb Mousse (see recipe, p.268) **125 kcal**
- 1 × 100ml serving Asda Triple Chocolate Dairy Ice Cream **101 kcal**
- 1 × 60g serving Tesco Healthy Living Banoffee Frozen Dessert **92 kcal**
- 1 × 100ml serving Wall's Soft Scoop Raspberry Ripple flavour ice cream **82 kcal** ☑
- 1 × 70g pot Marks & Spencer Count On Us Raspberry Mousse **80 kcal**
- 1 × 70g pot Marks & Spencer Count On Us Chocolate Mousse **80 kcal**
- 1 The Skinny Cow Triple Chocolate Stick **78 kcal** ☑
- 1 × 100ml serving Carte D'Or Lemon Sorbet **78 kcal**
- Tropical Sorbet (see recipe, p.267) **74 kcal** ☑
- 1 × 100ml serving Carte D'Or Light Vanilla ice cream **70 kcal**

■ 1 × 100ml serving Wall's Soft Scoop Light Vanilla flavour ice cream **62 kcal**

Fruit, meringues and jelly
■ Coffee and Apricot Roulade (see recipe, p.269) **108 kcal**
■ 150g fresh fruit salad plus 1 tsp low-fat yogurt **100 kcal**
■ Eton Mess: Break up 1 Marks & Spencer meringue basket and mix with 1 tbsp 0% fat Greek yogurt and 1 large chopped strawberry **99 kcal** ☑
■ 1 Marks & Spencer meringue nest filled with 1 tbsp 0% fat Greek yogurt and topped with 1 tbsp fresh raspberries or blueberries **90 kcal** ☑
■ 1 Marks & Spencer meringue basket filled with 1 tsp 0% fat Greek yogurt and topped with 1 slice pineapple, chopped **85 kcal** ☑
■ 1 × 120g pot Del Monte Fruitini Fruit Pieces in juice **71 kcal** ☑
■ 1 Hartley's Low Sugar Jelly plus 1 piece any fresh fruit **60 kcal**

Yogurts and fromage frais
■ 1 × 200g pot Müllerlight Apricot fat free yogurt **98 kcal**
■ 1 × 200g pot Müllerlight Wild Blueberry fat free yogurt **94 kcal**
■ 1 × 55g pot Asda Great Fruity Stuff fromage frais, any flavour **94 kcal** ☑
■ 1 × 125g pot Yeo Valley Organic Low Fat Raspberry Yogurt **94 kcal** ☑
■ 1 pot Tesco Healthy Living Lemon Cheesecake yogurt **90 kcal** ☑
■ 1 × 165g pot Müllerlight Vanilla Yogurt sprinkled with Dark Chocolate **86 kcal**
■ 1 × 125g pot Sainsbury's Be Good To Yourself Blueberry & Cranberry Fruit Yogurt **86 kcal**

- 1 × 150g Asda Good For You Rhubarb Yogurt **91 kcal** ☑
- 1 × 120g pot Danone Shape Fat Free Feel Fuller For Longer yogurt, any flavour **75 kcal** ☑

Puddings and cakes

- Crunchy Apple and Blackberry Pie (see recipe, p.273) **139 kcal** ☑
- Plum Tatin (see recipe, p.271) **107 kcal**
- 1 × 100ml serving Morrisons Absolutely Gorgeous Toffee Pecan Temptation **102 kcal**
- Banana Muffins (see recipe, p.270) **99 kcal**
- 1 Sainsbury's Lemon Cake Slice **97 kcal** ☑
- 1 Asda Good For You Lemon Slice **97 kcal** ☑
- 1 Asda Good for You Cherry Bakewell Slice **96 kcal**
- 1 Asda Good For You Chocolate Slice **95 kcal** ☑
- 1 Mr Kipling Delightful Apple Slice **91 kcal** ☑
- 1 Asda Good for You Carrot and Orange Cake Slice **77 kcal**
- 1 × 100g serving Tesco Healthy Eating Summer Fruits Pudding **72 kcal**
- 1 × ⅛ slice Soreen Lincolnshire Plum Fruit Loaf **65 kcal** ☑

TREATS

If you wish, you can combine one or more lower calorie treats. You can also save up your treats over seven days for a bigger treat or a special occasion.

HIGH-FAT TREATS FOR 100 KCAL OR LESS

All the following treats are more than 5 % fat.

Crisps

- 10 Pringles Lights Sour Cream & Onion flavour **99 kcal** ☑
- 1 × 21g bag Boots Shapers Salt & Vinegar Chipsticks **99 kcal** ☑

- 1 × 25g bag Walkers Baked Salt & Vinegar crisps **98 kcal** ☑
- 1 × 25g bag Jacob's Original Twiglets **96 kcal** ☑
- 1 × 18g bag Walkers Baked Wotsits Really Cheesy **95 kcal** ☑
- 1 × 19g bag Cheese & Onion Flavour Pom-Bear Teddy-shaped Potato Snacks **95 kcal** ☑
- 1 × 25g bag Walkers Squares Cheese & Onion Flavour Potato Snack **95 kcal** ☑
- 1 × 21g bag Golden Wonder Golden Lights Sour Cream & Onion crisps **94 kcal** ☑
- 1 × 21g bag Sainsbury's Be Good To Yourself 35% Less Fat Salt & Black Pepper Light & Crunchy Snacks **94 kcal** ☑
- 1 × 23g bag Walkers French Fries Ready Salted **94 kcal** ☑
- 1 × 25g bag Walkers Squares Ready Salted **94 kcal** ☑
- 1 × 24g bag Kettle Crispy Bakes Mild Cheese with Sweet Onion **91 kcal** ☑
- 1 × 18g bag Skips Prawn Cocktail snacks **89 kcal**
- 1 × 18g bag Walkers Quavers Cheese Flavour **87 kcal** ☑

Cereal bars and cakes
- 1 Cadbury Highlights Toffee Flavour Cake Bar **95 kcal** ☑
- 1 Mr Kipling Delightful Chocolate Cake Slice **95 kcal** ☑
- 1 Harvest Chewee White Choc Chip Cereal Bar **94 kcal** ☑
- 1 Kellogg's Special K Bar **90 kcal** ☑
- 1 Kellogg's Coco Pops Cereal & Milk Bar **85 kcal** ☑

Biscuits
- 2 Weight Watchers Raspberry & White Chocolate Cookies **98 kcal** ☑
- 2 Weight Watchers Double Choc Chip Cookies **98 kcal** ☑
- 3 Bahlsen Deloba biscuits **98 kcal** ☑
- 2 Sainsbury's Taste The Difference Belgian Chocolate Biscuit Thins **96 kcal**
- 3 Fox's Party Rings **93 kcal** ☑

- 1 Marks & Spencer All Butter Fruity Flapjack Cookie **95 kcal** ☑
- 2 McVitie's Jaffa Cakes **92 kcal** ☑
- 1 McVitie's Dark Chocolate HobNob **92 kcal** ☑
- 3 Rombouts Café Biscuits **92 kcal**
- 3 Cadbury Milk Chocolate Fingers **90 kcal** ☑
- 3 Lotus Original Caramelised Biscuits **90 kcal** ☑
- 1 Marks & Spencer Dutch Shortcake **90 kcal**
- 1 McVitie's Moments Chocolate Viennese Melt **90 kcal**
- 1 Tesco All Butter Traditional Scottish Shortbread Finger **90 kcal** ☑
- 4 Asda Rich Tea Fingers **88 kcal** ☑
- 1 Tesco Free From Golden Crunch biscuit **85 kcal** ☑
- 1 McVitie's Belgian Chocolate Chunk Boaster **86 kcal** ☑
- 1 Jammie Dodgers Original **83 kcal** ☑
- 1 McVitie's Milk Chocolate Mint Digestives **81 kcal**
- 1 Green & Black's Organic Chocolate Flapjack biscuit **80 kcal** ☑
- 4 Cadbury Snaps (any flavour) **80 kcal** ☑
- 1 McVitie's Light Milk Chocolate Digestive **78 kcal** ☑
- 1 Fox's Golden Crunch Creams **75 kcal** ☑

Sweets and chocolate
- 4 Bassetts Murray Mints **100 kcal** ☑
- 1 Boots Shapers Crispy Caramel Bar **99 kcal**
- 1 × 20g fun-size bag M & Ms **98 kcal**
- 1 fun-size Twix **98 kcal**
- 1 Tesco Value Choc Ice **95 kcal**
- 2 segments Terry's Chocolate Orange **90 kcal** ☑
- 6 Cadbury Mini Eggs **90 kcal** ☑
- 1 fun-size Mars Bar **88 kcal**
- 1 mini bag Nestlé Milkybar Buttons **87 kcal**
- 1 Thorntons Mini Caramel Shortcake **86 kcal** ☑

- 4 Werther's Original **84 kcal** ☑
- 2 Galaxy Mini Eggs **80 kcal** ☑
- 1 Ferrero Rocher **75 kcal** ☑
- 1 Thorntons Continental Chocolate **70 kcal** ☑

LOW-FAT TREATS FOR 100 KCAL OR LESS
All the following treats are less than 5% fat.

Sweet treats
- 2 Caxton Pink 'n' Whites **100 kcal** ☑
- 5 Bassetts Jelly Babies **100 kcal**
- 25 Jelly Belly Jelly Beans **100 kcal**
- 10 Maynards Wine Gums Light **100 kcal**
- 24 Skittles **97 kcal** ☑
- 1 × 28g treat bag Rowntree's Jelly Tots **96 kcal** ☑
- 4 Bassetts Liquorice Allsorts **91 kcal**
- 5 Starburst Twisted Chews **90 kcal** ☑
- 5 Haribo Tangfastics **85 kcal**

Savoury treats
- 1 × 25g bag Sainsbury's Be Good To Yourself Sea Salt & Cracked Black Pepper Pretzel Sticks **95 kcal**
- 1 × 25g pack Marks & Spencer Mini Salted Pretzels **94 kcal**
- 1 × 30g bag Ryvita Minis Salt & Vinegar **93 kcal**
- 1 × 25g bag Morrisons Eat Smart Sea Salt Pretzels **87 kcal**
- 1 × 25g bag Marks & Spencer Count On Us Sour Cream & Chive Baked Potato Crisps **85 kcal**
- 1 × 25g bag Marks & Spencer Count On Us Lightly Salted Baked Potato Crisps **85 kcal**
- 1 × 20g pack Asda Good For You Crispy Cracker Selection Hickory Smoked Barbecue Flavour **76 kcal**
- 1 × 20g pack Asda Good For You Crispy Cracker Selection Sun-Dried Tomato and Herb Flavour **76 kcal**

- 1 × 20g pack Asda Good For You Crispy Cracker Selection Thai Style Sweet Chilli Flavour **76 kcal**
- 1 × 25g bag Marks & Spencer Count On Us Smokey Bacon Potato Hoops **60 kcal**
- 1 × 18g pack Ryvita Limbos Cheese & Onion **63 kcal** ☑
- 1 × 18g pack Ryvita Limbos Smokey Bacon **63 kcal** ☑
- 1 × 18g pack Ryvita Limbos Salt & Vinegar **62 kcal** ☑

ALCOHOLIC DRINKS

In Phases 2 and 3 you are allowed an alcoholic drink each day up to 100 calories. Use Slimline and low-calorie mixers with spirits to keep the calories down. Here is a quick guide to calories.

Beer and cider (per 300ml/½ pint)
Bitter 91 kcal
Cider (dry) 100 kcal
Guinness 90 kcal
Lager 82 kcal

Brandy and liqueurs (per 25ml measure)
Brandy 50 kcal
Cointreau 78 kcal
Grand Marnier 78 kcal
Southern Comfort 81 kcal
Tia Maria 75 kcal

Spirits (per 25ml measure)
Bacardi 56 kcal
Gin 50 kcal
Rum 50 kcal
Vodka 50 kcal
Whisky 50 kcal

Vermouth (per 50ml measure)
Martini Extra Dry 48 kcal
Martini Rosso 70 kcal

Wine (per yellow Portion Pot®/125ml)
Champagne 95 kcal
Red wine 85 kcal
Rosé wine (medium) 89 kcal
White wine (dry) 83 kcal
White wine (medium) 93 kcal

Fortified wine (per 50ml measure)
Dry sherry 58 kcal
Sweet sherry 68 kcal
Port 79 kcal

9 Recipes

All these recipes are demonstrated by chef Dean Simpole-Clarke on www.rosemaryconley.tv

☑ means suitable for vegetarians
❄ means suitable for freezing

SOUPS

Broccoli and Leek Soup ☑❄

SERVES 4
Per serving
68 calories 1.9g fat
Preparation 10 minutes
Cooking time 20 minutes

4 leeks, sliced
2 garlic cloves, crushed
1 tsp chopped fresh thyme
1 litre vegetable stock
200g broccoli florets
2 tbsps chopped fresh parsley
200ml semi-skimmed milk
2 tbsps virtually fat free fromage frais
salt and freshly ground black pepper

1   Place the leeks, garlic and thyme in a large saucepan. Add the stock and bring to the boil. Simmer gently for 15 minutes.
2   Stir in the broccoli and parsley and continue cooking until the broccoli is tender.
3   Allow to cool a little, then pour into a liquidiser, add the milk and blend until smooth. Return to the saucepan to reheat, adding more seasoning if required.
4   Just before serving, remove from the heat and stir in the fromage frais.

Chicken, Mushroom and Lemon Soup

SERVES 4
Per serving
141 calories 2.7g fat
Preparation 10 minutes
Cooking 20 minutes

1 × 150g skinless chicken breast, cut into small pieces
2 celery sticks, finely chopped
2 leeks, finely chopped
2 garlic cloves, crushed
300ml vegetable stock
10g dried mushrooms
300ml semi-skimmed milk
1 tbsp cornflour
1 tsp fine lemon zest
1 tbsp chopped fresh parsley
2 tbsps low-fat yogurt
fresh chives to serve

TIP *Dried mushrooms add a strong flavour to this creamy soup*

1 Preheat a large non-stick pan, then dry-fry the chicken, celery, leeks and garlic for 2–3 minutes. Stir in the stock and mushrooms and boil until the mushrooms are soft.
2 Pour the milk into the soup and simmer gently for 10–15 minutes.
3 Mix the cornflour with a little cold water and stir into the soup, along with the lemon zest, to allow the soup to thicken.
4 Once the soup has thickened, stir in the parsley. Just before serving, remove from the heat and stir in the yogurt. Garnish with a few chives.

Chicken Noodle Soup ❄

SERVES 4
Per serving
170 calories 1.4g fat
Preparation 25 minutes
Cooking 30 minutes

200g lean chicken breast (no skin), cut into strips
3 baby leeks, finely chopped
1 garlic clove, crushed
2 tsps ground coriander
½ tsp ground turmeric
1 small fresh green chilli, chopped
seeds from 4 crushed cardamom pods
600ml vegetable stock
100g fine rice noodles
2 tbsps chopped fresh basil
50g shredded fresh watercress
freshly ground black pepper

1   Preheat a non-stick wok or frying pan, then dry-fry the
    chicken until lightly browned on all sides and season with
    black pepper. Place to one side.
2   Place the leeks, garlic, spices, vegetable stock and rice
    noodles in a large saucepan and bring to a gentle simmer.
3   When the noodles are cooked, add the chicken to the pan
    and stir in the basil and watercress. Serve straight away.

TIP *Using rice noodles makes
this a gluten-free dish*

CHICKEN AND TURKEY

Chinese Chicken Kebabs

SERVES 2
Per serving
204 calories 1.6g fat
Preparation 10 minutes
Marinating 1 hour
Cooking 20 minutes

TIP *Marinate the kebabs overnight for maximum flavour*

2 medium-sized skinless chicken breasts
1 red pepper, diced
1 small can water chestnuts
1 tbsp dark brown sugar
1 tbsp cider vinegar
1 tsp finely chopped fresh ginger
1 tbsp tomato purée
salt and freshly ground black pepper
chopped spring onions to serve

1   Cut the chicken into chunks. Thread the chicken, red pepper and water chestnuts on to 4 wooden or metal skewers and place on a baking tray. Season with salt and black pepper.
2   Mix together the remaining ingredients, then drizzle over the kebabs. Leave the kebabs for at least an hour to allow them to absorb the marinade.
3   Cook the kebabs in a health grill for 10 minutes or under a preheated hot grill for 8–10 minutes each side.
4   Transfer to serving plates and garnish with spring onion.

Barbecued Garlic Chicken

SERVES 4
Per serving
155 calories 1.4g fat
Preparation 10 minutes
Marinating 1 hour
Cooking 30 minutes

4 skinless chicken breasts (400g total)
salt and freshly ground black pepper

for the marinade
2 tbsps sweet chilli sauce
2 tbsps runny honey
1 tbsp Worcestershire sauce
2 garlic cloves, peeled and chopped
1 red onion, finely chopped
pinch of fennel seeds

1   Combine the marinade ingredients in a mixing bowl.
2   Season the chicken breasts with salt and black pepper and
    place in the bottom of an ovenproof dish. Spoon the
    marinade over the chicken and leave to marinate for at
    least 1 hour.
3   Cook under a preheated grill or on
    a preheated barbecue for 25–30   **TIP** *For maximum*
    minutes until cooked through to   *flavour, leave the*
    the centre.   *chicken to marinate*
4   Serve straight away with a   *overnight in the*
    selection of fresh vegetables or   *refrigerator*
    salads.

Chicken Shaslik

SERVES 4
Per serving
170 calories 2.4g fat
Preparation 15 minutes
Cooking 30 minutes

TIP *Mix together some chopped fresh coriander and a little low-fat yogurt to make a simple sauce to serve alongside this dish*

4 skinless chicken breasts (400g total)
1 red pepper, cut into chunks
1 green pepper, cut into chunks
1 red onion, cut into chunks
2 garlic cloves, crushed
1 × 2cm piece fresh ginger, peeled and chopped
1 tsp ground turmeric
2 tsps ground coriander
2 tsps tandoori powder
1 × 400g can chopped tomatoes
1–2 tsps vegetable stock powder
salt and freshly ground black pepper

1   Preheat a non-stick wok.
2   Chop the chicken breasts into chunks.
3   Dry-fry the peppers and onion in the wok for 2–3 minutes.
    Add the chicken, garlic and ginger and cook until the
    chicken is sealed. Stir in the spices and cook for a further
    minute. Finally, add the tomatoes and stock powder, then
    reduce the heat and simmer gently for 10 minutes before
    serving.
4   For a dinner option, serve with 1 blue Portion Pot® (55g
    uncooked weight) or 1 red Portion Pot® (144g cooked
    weight) basmati rice per person.

Southern Fried Turkey

SERVES 2
Per serving
354 calories 6.2 g fat
Preparation 10 minutes
Cooking 30 minutes

4 thin turkey escalopes (320g total)
1 egg, beaten

for the coating
4 tbsps granary breadcrumbs
1 garlic clove, crushed
1 tsp paprika
1 tsp jerk seasoning
1 tbsp chopped fresh chives
salt and freshly ground black pepper

1   Preheat the oven to 200C, 400F, Gas Mark 6.
2   Mix together the breadcrumbs, garlic and seasonings and
    transfer to a non-stick baking tray. Place in the oven for 10
    minutes until the breadcrumbs are lightly toasted.
3   Dip the turkey escalopes in the beaten egg and then the
    breadcrumbs and place on a non-stick baking tray. Bake in
    the oven for 25–30 minutes until cooked through.
4   Serve with fresh vegetables or salad.

Turkey and Mango Samosas

SERVES 4
Per serving
227 calories 6.1g fat
Preparation 20 minutes
Cooking 15–20 minutes

TIP *These tasty pastry triangles also make ideal party food*

2 baby leeks, finely chopped
1 garlic clove, crushed
200g turkey mince
1–2 tsps vegetable stock powder
1 tbsp chopped fresh mint
1 tbsp mango chutney
4 sheets filo pastry
olive oil spray
salt and freshly ground black pepper

1   Preheat the oven to 200C, 400F, Gas Mark 6.
2   Preheat a non-stick frying pan, then dry-fry the leeks and garlic for 2–3 minutes until soft. Add the turkey and continue cooking for 5 minutes. Stir in the stock powder, mint and chutney and mix well. Remove from the heat and allow to cool.
3   Place the filo sheets on a chopping board. Cut each sheet into 3 lengthways, then lightly spray with oil spray. Place a dessertspoon of turkey mixture at each end of the strips, fold the pastry over diagonally to enclose the meat in a triangle, then transfer to a baking tray and spray again with oil.
4   Bake in the oven for 15–20 minutes until golden brown. Serve with fresh vegetables or salad.

BEEF, LAMB AND PORK

Lamb Medallions with Blackcurrant Sauce

SERVES 4
Per serving
200 calories 10.8g fat
Preparation 10 minutes
Marinating 30 minutes
Cooking 15 minutes

TIP *Lamb medallions are the leanest cut of lamb available and they can be cooked and eaten pink*

8 lamb medallions, all visible fat removed
1 tbsp blackcurrant jelly
2 garlic cloves, crushed
150ml vegetable stock
1 tbsp chopped fresh mint
salt and freshly ground black pepper

1   Place the lamb in a shallow dish and season with salt and pepper.
2   In a small saucepan heat together the blackcurrant jelly, garlic and vegetable stock for 2 minutes until the garlic is soft. Allow to cool, then stir in the mint.
3   Drizzle the sauce over the lamb and leave to marinate for 30 minutes.
4   Preheat the grill to high. Place the lamb on a baking tray and cook under the hot grill for 4–5 minutes each side, turning regularly. Serve hot.
5   For a dinner option, serve with 100g boiled new potatoes (with skins) and unlimited vegetables per person.

Cheesy Cottage Pie ❄

SERVES 4
Per serving
409 calories 16.3g fat
Preparation 10 minutes
Cooking 40 minutes

300g celeriac, peeled and chopped
300g sweet potato, peeled and chopped
500g lean beef mince
1 red onion, finely chopped
2 garlic cloves, crushed
2 tsps vegetable stock powder
3 carrots (300g total), peeled and diced
1 tbsp chopped fresh herbs
1 tbsp gravy granules
2 tbsps skimmed milk
50g Rosemary Conley low-fat Mature Cheese, grated
salt and freshly ground black pepper

1   Preheat the oven to 200C, 400F, Gas Mark 6. Preheat a
    non-stick pan.
2   Boil the celeriac and potatoes together in a saucepan of
    water until soft.
3   Meanwhile, dry-fry the mince in the
    non-stick pan until lightly browned.
    Tip the mince into a sieve to drain
    off the fat, then return it to the
    pan, add the onion, garlic and stock
    powder and cook for 3–4 minutes.
    [continued]

TIP *Using half*
sweet potatoes and
mashed celeriac
lowers the Gi rating
of this dish

4 Add the carrots and herbs to the pan, then pour in 300ml water and bring to a gentle simmer. Add the gravy granules and continue to simmer for 20 minutes to allow the sauce to thicken. Check the seasoning, then transfer to an ovenproof dish.

5 Drain the celeriac and potatoes and mash well, adding the skimmed milk and seasoning with salt and black pepper. Spread the potato mixture over the meat and vegetables and smooth over the top, using a fork. Finally sprinkle the cheese on top.

6 Bake in the top of the oven for 20 minutes until golden brown.

Lamb and Mushroom Goulash ❄

SERVES 4
Per serving
332 calories 10.6g fat
Preparation 10 minutes
Cooking 70 minutes

2 red onions, diced
2 garlic cloves, crushed
450g lean diced lamb
1 tbsp flour
2 tsps paprika
1.2 litres meat stock
10g dried wild mushrooms
2 tbsps tomato purée
450g small new potatoes
2 celery sticks, chopped
200g button mushrooms
1 tbsp mixed herbs (e.g. parsley, thyme, chives)
salt and freshly ground black pepper

TIP *Choose lean diced lamb and remove all visible traces of fat before cooking*

1 Preheat a non-stick pan, then dry-fry the onions and garlic until the onion starts to brown.
2 Add the lamb to the pan, season with salt and black pepper and cook until sealed. Sprinkle the flour and paprika over and cook out for 1 minute, then gradually stir in the meat stock.
3 Add the remaining ingredients, then cover and simmer gently for 1 hour until the meat is tender. Serve with green vegetables.

Wine Braised Pork Slices ❄

SERVES 4
Per serving
191 calories 4.5g fat
Preparation 10 minutes
Cooking 25 minutes

1 red onion, diced
2 garlic cloves, crushed
4 lean pork slices (400g total), all visible fat removed
100g chestnut mushrooms, sliced
2 tsps ground coriander
75ml red wine
1–2 tsps vegetable stock powder
2 × 400g cans chopped tomatoes
salt and freshly ground black pepper
fresh parsley to garnish

1 Preheat a non-stick pan, then dry-fry the onion and garlic
   until the onion is lightly browned.
2 Add the pork slices to the pan and cook until sealed,
   seasoning with salt and black pepper. Stir in the
   mushrooms and coriander and cook, mixing well, before
   adding the vegetable stock powder, wine and tomatoes.
   Cover and simmer for 20 minutes until the sauce has
   reduced.
3 Transfer to serving plates and garnish with fresh parsley.
4 For a dinner option, serve with 115g boiled new potatoes
   (with skins) per person and additional other vegetables of
   your choice.

Ham, Leek and Sweet Potato Pie ✳

SERVES 4
Per serving
303 calories 3.5g fat
Preparation 10 minutes
Cooking 20 minutes

900g sweet potatoes, peeled
2 leeks, washed and sliced
100g thin ham, chopped
2–3 tbsps semi-skimmed milk
100g low-fat mature cheese
pinch of nutmeg
4 medium-sized tomatoes
salt and freshly ground black pepper

1 Preheat the oven to 200C, 400F, Gas Mark 6.
2 Boil the potatoes in a large pan of salted water until soft.
   Drain the potatoes, then mash them, adding the leeks, ham
   and milk.
3 Using a wooden spoon, fold in half the cheese along with
   the nutmeg and season to taste with salt and black pepper,
   then pile the potato mixture into an ovenproof dish.
4 Slice the tomatoes and arrange on
   top of the potatoes. Sprinkle with the
   remaining cheese and bake in the
   oven for 20 minutes or until golden
   brown.
5 Serve with fresh vegetables
   (excluding potatoes) or salad.

TIP *If you slice
the leeks very fine,
they will not need
pre-cooking
before adding to
the potatoes*

Brunch Pitta

MAKES 2
Per pitta
291 calories 6.1g fat
Preparation 5 minutes
Cooking 10 minutes

2 pitta breads (max. 200 calories each)
4 rashers lean back bacon
2 tomatoes, sliced in half
2 large mushrooms (50g total), sliced
1 tbsp tomato ketchup
freshly ground black pepper

1 Preheat a health grill or conventional grill to high.
2 Cook the bacon, tomatoes and mushrooms in the health
   grill for 4–5 minutes or place in a grill tray or on a baking
   tray and cook under the conventional grill for 4–5 minutes
   each side, turning regularly. Remove and keep warm.
3 Warm the pittas in the health grill or under the
   conventional grill for 1 minute until puffed up, then split
   them in half and spread the insides with the ketchup.
   Divide the bacon, tomatoes and mushrooms between the
   2 pitta breads, then cut each pitta bread in half and serve.

FISH AND SEAFOOD

Black Bean Prawns

SERVES 4
Per serving
135 calories 1.7g fat
Preparation 10 minutes
Cooking 10 minutes

2 red onions, finely sliced
2 garlic cloves, crushed
1 green and 1 red pepper, deseeded and sliced
110g chestnut mushrooms, sliced
200g fresh peeled prawns
100g Chinese cabbage, shredded
150ml black bean sauce
2 tbsps low-salt soy sauce
1 tbsp maple syrup
zest and juice of 1 lemon
freshly ground black pepper

1   Preheat a non-stick wok, then dry-fry the onions and garlic
    over a high heat for 3–4 minutes, seasoning well with black
    pepper. Add the peppers and mushrooms and continue
    cooking for 1–2 minutes, then stir in the prawns, cabbage
    and the black bean and soy sauces and toss well.
2   Once the prawns have changed colour, add the remaining
    ingredients, toss well and heat through before serving.
3   For a dinner option, serve with 1 blue Portion Pot® (55g
    uncooked weight) or 1 red Portion Pot® (144g cooked
    weight) basmati rice per person.

Prawn Saag

SERVES 4
Per serving
118 calories 1.3g fat
Preparation 10 minutes
Cooking 20 minutes

TIP *This sauce also works well with chicken or, for a vegetarian version, you can substitute Quorn pieces*

175g cooked shelled prawns
1 red onion, finely chopped
2 garlic cloves, crushed
1 green pepper, deseeded and finely diced
1 × 400g can chopped tomatoes
300ml tomato passata
1 green chilli, seeded and finely chopped
200g fresh spinach
salt and freshly ground black pepper
chopped fresh coriander to garnish

1 Rinse the prawns well under cold running water.
2 Preheat a non-stick frying pan, then dry-fry the onion for
   2–3 minutes until soft.
3 Add the garlic and green pepper to the pan and cook for
   2–3 minutes. Stir in the tomatoes, tomato passata and
   chilli, and bring the sauce to a gentle simmer, then add
   the prawns and the spinach and heat through.
4 Season to taste with salt and black pepper before serving
   and garnish with the coriander.
5 For a dinner option, serve with 1 green Portion Pot® (170g)
   cooked egg noodles or 1 blue Portion Pot® (55g uncooked
   weight) or 1 red Portion Pot® (144g cooked weight)
   basmati rice per person.

Singapore Noodles with Prawns

SERVES 4
Per serving
212 calories 3.4g fat
Preparation 10 minutes
Cooking 20 minutes

110g fine noodles
2 leeks, finely sliced
2 garlic cloves, crushed
1 red pepper, deseeded and finely sliced
1 × 5cm piece lemongrass, finely chopped
175g mangetout
3 tbsps pineapple juice
1 tbsp soy sauce
225g peeled uncooked prawns
225g beansprouts
salt and freshly ground black pepper

1 Cook the noodles in boiling water, then drain.
2 Preheat a non-stick wok, then dry-fry the leeks and garlic
   until soft. Add the red pepper, lemongrass, mangetout,
   pineapple juice and soy sauce and toss well together. Stir
   in the prawns and cook until they change colour. Stir in the
   beansprouts and drained noodles and combine well.
   Serve hot.
3 For a lunch option, serve with a
   crisp salad.

TIP *For a vegetarian option, use Quorn pieces instead of prawns*

VEGETARIAN

Leek and Sage Meatballs with Pasta ✔

SERVES 4
Per serving
390 calories 7.7g fat
Preparation 10 minutes
Cooking 25 minutes

500g Quorn mince
2 leeks, finely chopped
1 garlic clove, crushed
1 tbsp finely chopped sage
1 tbsp grainy mustard
1 tsp vegetable stock powder
1 egg, beaten
500g tomato passata
1 tbsp chopped fresh basil, plus extra for the garnish
1 tsp runny honey
200g (dry weight) pasta shapes
freshly ground black pepper
10g low-fat mature cheese to serve

1 Place the Quorn mince in a mixing bowl. Add the leeks, garlic, sage, mustard and stock powder and mix well. Mix in the beaten egg, then divide the mixture into 20 golfball-sized balls.

TIP *As a variation you can substitute beef, chicken or pork mince for the Quorn*

2   Preheat a non-stick pan, then dry-fry the meatballs,
    browning them on all sides. Add the tomato passata, 1 tbsp
    of basil and the honey and season with black pepper.
3   Meanwhile, cook the pasta in a pan of boiling water, then
    drain well and transfer to warmed serving bowls.
4   Spoon the sauce on top and garnish with the remaining
    basil and a little grated low-fat mature cheese.

Amazing Inch Loss Salad ☑

SERVES 1
61 calories 1.2g fat

4 cherry tomatoes, halved
4 thick slices cucumber, chopped
3 button mushrooms, halved
1 celery stick, chopped
½ green pepper, sliced
25g fresh beansprouts (optional)
25g mixed salad leaves
1 dsp (10ml) fat-free dressing

1   Mix all the salad vegetables together and arrange on top of
    the salad leaves.
2   Drizzle with the fat-free dressing and serve as a side salad.

Garlic Mushroom Pasta ☑

SERVES 4
Per serving
270 calories 4.5g fat
Preparation 10 minutes
Cooking 20 minutes

200g (dry weight) pasta shapes
1 vegetable stock cube
3 baby leeks (240g total), finely sliced
2 garlic cloves, crushed
200g button mushrooms
a few chilli flakes
200g Philadelphia Extra Light soft cheese
100ml semi-skimmed milk
1 tbsp chopped fresh basil
salt and freshly ground black pepper
olive oil spray

1   Cook the pasta in a pan of water containing the stock cube.
2   Preheat a non-stick pan, then dry-fry the leeks, garlic and
    mushrooms for 2–3 minutes in a little olive oil spray, taking
    care not to burn the garlic.
3   Add the chilli flakes and cheese, then season with salt and
    black pepper and cook for 8–10 minutes, adding enough
    milk to make a coating sauce.
    Finally, stir in the basil.
4   Drain the pasta well, return it to
    the pan, then add the sauce
    and toss well. Serve straight
    away with a small salad.

TIP *You can also serve
this mushroom sauce
with warm pitta slices
instead of pasta*

Roasted Pepper Pasta ☑

SERVES 4
Per serving
247 calories 1.5g fat
Preparation 20 minutes
Cooking 25 minutes

TIP *Add a pinch of dried chilli flakes to spice up the sauce*

2 long red peppers (approx. 300g total)
200g (dry weight) pasta shapes
1 vegetable stock cube
1 red onion, finely sliced
2 garlic cloves, crushed
1 × 500g pack tomato passata
salt and freshly ground black pepper
olive oil spray
chopped fresh basil to garnish

1   Preheat the oven to 200C, 400F, Gas Mark 6.
2   Put the peppers on a non-stick baking tray, spray lightly with olive oil and season with salt and pepper.
3   Place the peppers in the oven for 15–20 minutes until their skins start to lift away. Remove from the oven, cover the peppers completely with clear food wrap and leave to cool until the skins come away. Peel and chop the peppers and remove the seeds.
4   Cook the pasta in a large saucepan of boiling water with the stock cube.
5   Meanwhile, preheat a non-stick pan, then dry-fry the onion and garlic until soft. Add the peppers and passata and bring to a gentle simmer.
6   Drain the pasta thoroughly, arrange on warmed plates, pour the pepper sauce over and garnish with the basil.
7   Serve with a large salad tossed in fat-free dressing.

Quorn and Rice Bake ☑

SERVES 4
Per serving
339 calories 5g fat
Preparation 15 minutes
Cooking 25 minutes

TIP *Keep the vegetables quite chunky to add texture to the finished dish*

2 medium red onions, cut into wedges
2 garlic cloves, crushed
2 celery sticks, chopped
1 red pepper, deseeded and diced
1 red chilli, sliced
4 Quorn fillets, cut into chunks
225g (dry weight) basmati rice
2 tsps vegetable stock powder
1 × 400g can chopped tomatoes
600ml water
salt and freshly ground black pepper
chopped fresh parsley to garnish

1   Preheat a non-stick frying pan.
2   Dry-fry the onions in the non-stick pan until lightly
     browned, then add the garlic, celery, pepper, chilli and
     Quorn. Stir in the rice, stock powder and tomatoes, and
     pour in sufficient water (approx. 600ml) to cover the rice.
     Bring to the boil, then reduce the heat and simmer gently
     for 20 minutes until the liquid has been absorbed and the
     rice is cooked.
3   Season to taste with black pepper before serving and
     garnish with the chopped parsley.
4   For a dinner option, serve with unlimited vegetables
     (excluding potatoes).

Bombay Rice ✓ ❄

SERVES 4
Per serving
212 calories 2.1g fat
Preparation 10 minutes
Cooking 20 minutes

1 red onion, finely chopped
2 garlic cloves, crushed
1 red pepper, deseeded and diced
160g (dry weight) brown basmati rice
1 tbsp fajita mix powder
110g frozen peas
1 small red chilli, finely sliced
500ml vegetable stock
2 tbsps chopped fresh parsley
salt and freshly ground black pepper

1   Preheat a large non-stick pan, then dry-fry the onion, garlic and red pepper until soft.
2   Add the rice, fajita mix powder, peas and chilli, then pour in the stock and cook over a high heat until the rice is cooked and has absorbed all the liquid.
3   Just before serving sprinkle with the parsley. Serve with salad.

TIP *For a main dish, add a few cooked vegetables or stir in some cooked prawns*

Stir-Fried Rice Noodles ☑

SERVES 1
Per serving
186 calories 1.4g fat
Preparation 10 minutes
Cooking 10 minutes

30g rice noodles
2 baby leeks, finely sliced
½ garlic clove, crushed
½ yellow pepper, deseeded and sliced
2 baby courgettes, sliced
50g chestnut mushrooms, sliced
2 tsps soy sauce
1 tsp rice vinegar
squeeze of fresh lemon juice
freshly ground black pepper

1   Cook the rice noodles in boiling water and drain.
2   Preheat a non-stick wok, then add the leeks and garlic and
    dry-fry over a high heat for 3–4 minutes, seasoning well
    with black pepper. Add the yellow pepper, courgettes and
    mushrooms and continue cooking for 1–2 minutes. Stir in
    the cooked noodles along with the remaining ingredients
    and toss well together. Serve straight away.

TIP *For a fresh herb flavour, add some chopped
coriander to the noodles as you drain them*

Cauliflower Bhaji ☑

SERVES 4
Per serving
107 calories 2.2g fat
Preparation 10 minutes
Cooking 20 minutes

2 red onions, chopped
2 garlic cloves, crushed
1 red pepper, deseeded and diced
1 cauliflower (300g), broken into florets
1 tbsp medium curry powder
2–3 curry leaves
1 green chilli, finely chopped
1 × 400g can chopped tomatoes
1–2 tsps vegetable stock powder
1 tbsp tomato purée
salt and freshly ground black pepper

1   Preheat a large non-stick pan, then dry-fry the onions and garlic for 1–2 minutes until soft. Add the red pepper, cauliflower and curry powder and cook for a further 5 minutes.
2   Stir in the remaining ingredients, add sufficient water to cook the cauliflower, and simmer gently for 10 minutes until the cauliflower is cooked, topping up with a little extra water if required.

TIP *Serve this simple curry as a side dish with meat or fish or as a vegetarian main course with rice*

Greek Salad Wrap ✔

MAKES 2
Per wrap
279 calories 6.6g fat
Preparation 5 minutes
Cooking 1–2 minutes

2 tortilla wraps
2 tbsps Philadelphia Extra Light soft cheese
4 fresh mint leaves, chopped
few rocket leaves
2 tomatoes, sliced
½ red pepper, deseeded and finely chopped
thinly sliced cucumber
freshly ground black pepper

1   Preheat a health grill or conventional grill to high.
2   Spread the tortillas with the cheese. Sprinkle the mint
    leaves over and add the rocket leaves, tomatoes, red
    pepper and cucumber, then season with black pepper. Roll
    up the tortillas, folding the ends in.
3   Place the wraps on the health grill or under the
    conventional grill for 1–2 minutes. Serve warm.

TIP *Pep up these wraps with some pickled chillies*

DESSERTS

Tropical Sorbet ❄

SERVES 8
Per serving
74 calories 0.1 g fat
Preparation 20 minutes
Cooking 10 minutes
Freezing 7 hours

110g caster sugar
1 ripe mango, peeled and sliced
2 passion fruit, seeds removed
1 papaya, peeled and seeds removed
zest and juice of 1 lemon
1 egg white

1   In a saucepan dissolve the sugar in 300ml water and bring
    to the boil, then remove from the heat and allow to cool.
2   Place all the fruit in a liquidiser and blend until smooth.
3   Mix the fruit with the cooled syrup, add the lemon zest and
    juice and pour into a shallow freezer container. Freeze for
    about 3 hours until mushy.
4   Whisk the egg white until stiff and
    fold into the loosened sorbet.
    Refreeze for 4 hours or overnight
    until firm.
5   Serve in chilled glasses with
    additional fruit if desired.

TIP *Remove the
sorbet from the
freezer 5 minutes
before required to
allow it to soften
before serving*

Strawberry and Rhubarb Mousse

SERVES 6
Per serving
125 calories 2.9g fat
Preparation 20 minutes

1 × 410g can Carnation Light evaporated milk
340g fresh strawberries, hulled
6 sticks rhubarb (900g total), chopped
2 tbsps ginger wine or ginger ale
1 tbsp caster sugar
6 gelatine leaves
pinch of sugar
2 egg whites

1   Chill the Carnation milk overnight in the refrigerator or place in the freezer for 30 minutes until cold.
2   Using an electric whisk, whisk the milk until thick and creamy.
3   Reserve 4 strawberries and place the remainder in a saucepan. Add the rhubarb, ginger wine or ale and caster sugar and bring to the boil.
4   Soften the gelatine in cold water, then squeeze out the water, add the gelatine to the pan and stir well until dissolved.
5   Pour the fruit mixture into a blender and blend until smooth. If you wish, you can strain the mixture through a sieve to remove the seeds.
6   In a separate bowl, whisk the egg whites until stiff, adding a pinch of sugar. Fold the egg whites into the chilled, whisked milk, then fold in the strawberry purée.
7   Pour into serving glasses, decorate with the reserved strawberries and chill until ready to serve.

Coffee and Apricot Roulade

SERVES 8
Per serving
108 calories 0.2g fat
Preparation 5 minutes
Cooking 20 minutes

4 egg whites
175g caster sugar
2 tsps instant coffee granules
4 tbsps 0% fat Greek yogurt
3 fresh apricots, chopped

1   Preheat the oven to 150C, 300F, Gas Mark 2.
2   In a clean, dry bowl, whisk the egg whites to stiff peaks,
    then fold in the caster sugar a dessertspoon at a time, at
    10-second intervals.
3   Pour the mixture onto a baking tray lined with baking
    parchment. Sprinkle the coffee granules over, then swirl the
    granules into the mixture.
4   Bake in the oven for 20 minutes, then remove the meringue
    from the oven, turn out onto foil and allow to cool.
5   When the meringue is cool, spread with the Greek yogurt,
    top with the apricots, then roll up lengthways to form a
    roulade.

Banana Muffins

MAKES 6
Per muffin
99 calories 3.9g fat
Preparation 10 minutes
Cooking 20 minutes

TIP *Store these gluten-free muffins in an airtight container and keep for up to 2 days*

3 tbsps Alpro cream alternative
1 tsp cider vinegar
2 tbsps golden caster sugar
1 × 100g banana
lemon juice
2 eggs, beaten
2 tbsps gluten-free flour
1 tsp gluten-free baking powder
1 tbsp icing sugar
speck of turmeric

1. Preheat the oven to 150C, 350F, Gas Mark 4.
2. Line a 6-hole muffin tin with papers. Whisk together the Alpro, vinegar and sugar until light and fluffy. Cut 6 thin slices from the banana (reserve the remainder) and place in a little lemon juice. Mash the remaining banana and add to the mix. Add the eggs, flour and baking powder, blending well together. Spoon into the papers and bake in the oven for 20 minutes.
3. Remove from oven and allow to cool. Mix together the icing sugar with the turmeric, add a little boiling water and stir until smooth. Pour onto the cakes and top with the reserved banana slices.

Plum Tatin

SERVES 6
Per serving
107 calories 0.8g fat
Preparation 10 minutes
Cooking 30 minutes

6 dark plums
2 tbsps caster sugar
4 sheets filo pastry
low-calorie spray oil

1   Preheat the oven to 200C, 400F, Gas Mark 6. Preheat a
    non-stick frying pan.
2   Remove the stones from the plums, place the stoned plums
    in the hot pan, add the sugar and cook over a low heat until
    the sugar starts to colour. Remove the plums from the pan
    and place in the base of a silicone cake mould.
3   Add 2 tbsps of water to the pan (be careful of the steam as
    the water comes into contact with the hot sugar). Heat
    until the sugar is dissolved, then pour over the plums. Layer
    the filo pastry sheets on top, spraying in between the layers
    with a little spray oil.
4   Bake in the oven for 15–20
    minutes until golden in colour,
    then remove from the oven and
    allow to cool slightly before
    turning out onto a serving plate.
    Serve hot or cold with
    low-fat yogurt.

TIP *Choose firm
plums that will stand
up to cooking – avoid
over-ripe ones as
they will become soft
and lose their shape*

Frozen Berry Smoothie

SERVES 1
Per serving
181 calories 0.7g fat
Preparation 5 minutes

50g frozen blueberries
50g frozen raspberries
1 small banana
200ml apple juice

1   Place all the ingredients into a
    smoothie maker or liquidiser and
    blend until smooth.
2   Serve as a speedy breakfast or
    dessert.

TIP *If the mixture is
too thick, add a little
boiling water to thin
it down*

Amazing Meringue Sundae

SERVES 1
73 calories 0.2g fat

1 meringue basket (approx. 50 kcal)
1 tsp Total 0% fat Greek Yoghurt
4 sliced strawberries (or 50g raspberries or 40g blueberries)

1   Fill the meringue basket with the yogurt and top with
    berries of your choice.

Crunchy Apple and Blackberry Pie

SERVES 4
Per serving
139 calories 0.8g fat
Preparation 15 minutes
Cooking 20 minutes

600g cooking apples
2 tsps salt
200g blackberries
2 tbsps golden caster sugar
2 sheets (100g total) filo pastry
pinch of mixed spice
low-calorie cooking oil spray

1   Preheat the oven to 150C, 300F, Gas Mark 2.
2   Peel and slice the apples into a bowl of salted water. Rinse
    well and place in the bottom of an ovenproof dish. Scatter
    the blackberries over and sprinkle with 1 tbsp of the sugar.
3   Cut the filo pastry sheets in half to give 4 sheets. Spray a
    sheet lightly with oil spray and place on top of the fruit,
    scrunching it up to give a wrinkled effect. Repeat with the
    other sheets, until the fruit is covered.
4   Spray the top sheet lightly with
    oil spray, sprinkle with the
    remaining sugar and dust with
    the mixed spice.
5   Bake in the centre of the oven for
    20 minutes until crisp and
    golden. Serve hot or cold with
    low-fat yogurt.

TIP *Slicing the apples
into salted water and
then rinsing them
prevents them from
turning brown as well
as adding flavour*

10 The Amazing Inch Loss maintenance toning programme

If you've followed this Amazing Inch Loss Plan on a day-by-day basis and done the exercises with me on www.rosemaryconley.tv, to accompany this book, you should have seen a dramatic improvement in your shape and noticed an increase in your overall muscle strength.

This maintenance toning workout is super-effective and really quite advanced. You should only undertake it if you have progressed through the 28-day exercise programme, from my original *Amazing Inch Loss Plan* book or on www.rosemaryconley.tv where I demonstrate each day's exercises. If not, you will probably find the exercises here too hard and then you may get disheartened and give up, which would be a terrible shame. However, if you have completed the 28-day programme, you will be able to do these exercises very easily and maintain your new fit and healthy figure.

Personally, for my own maintenance workout, I do the exercises in the toning sections of my Real Results DVD, which are similar to the ones on the following pages. It enables my muscles to stay strong and all of my joints to remain fit and healthy so that I don't ache anywhere or find moving about difficult. It's a great all-round, advanced toning programme so

I hope you will enjoy it, too, once you've reached a certain level of fitness.

You may also be interested in participating in my nightly fitness challenge on Twitter. You can follow me on Twitter@rosemaryconley, and each evening I post a fitness challenge which takes only a few minutes to do, but that little bit of extra strength training or aerobic activity can make a difference over time.

For maximum benefits, practise this toning programme three times a week. If you do the exercises in the order shown, with the recommended number of repetitions, you will maintain the tremendous benefits that you have already enjoyed. It's important to warm up your body first, as this will enhance your performance and enable you to perform the exercises more effectively. Likewise, always do the stretches at the end (see page 288) as these release the toxins that can build up during the exercise, which will prevent muscle soreness later. The whole routine takes no longer than 10 minutes so it's worth warming up and cooling down properly.

This workout is not featured on rosemaryconley.tv but the exercises are featured in my Real Results DVD. The toning programmes in my Real Results DVD are incredibly effective. There are four toning workouts in all – two of which take 10 minutes and two of which take fewer than five minutes. The DVD also contains an extremely effective aerobic routine. This is what Alison Mowe, one of the followers of the DVD, wrote about her progress:

'I have worked out every day with your Real Results DVD as I find it absolutely fantastic. I love the workouts, the music, and the girls look wonderful. It really is a pleasure to get up at 6.30 a.m. and do the routines. Even my 10-year-old daughter has had a go and she loves it. So thank you for a fantastic DVD.'

Warm-up

1 Knee lifts with pull-downs
Stand upright with hands above head and tummy pulled in. Lift alternate knees and as you lift, pull your arms down to either side of the knees. Keep your tummy in and your back straight and continue for 1 minute.

2 Pretend skipping
Imagine you are holding a skipping rope. Begin a small bounce on the spot as you pretend to turn the rope. You can turn around in a circle and even do some fancy arm work such as figure 8s.

3 Ski swings
Stand tall and lift both arms overhead, pulling your tummy in. Now swing your arms down and past your thighs as you bend your knees and hips. Keep your back straight and keep looking forward. Come up again and repeat the ski swings for 1 minute.

4 March on spot with tummy pull-ins
Stand tall and march on the spot, letting your arms swing naturally. Really pull your tummy in tight for 10 steps and then relax it for 10 steps.

Ten-minute tone-up – advanced

1 Shoulder shaper (3 × 12 reps)
Stand tall with your tummy in, feet apart, knees slightly bent, arms by your sides and a handweight or water bottle in each hand Ⓐ. Now breathe in and, as you breathe out, lift both arms out to the sides at shoulder height Ⓑ. Keep your arms slightly bent and in front of your body with palms facing down. Do 12 reps, then rest before doing another 2 sets.

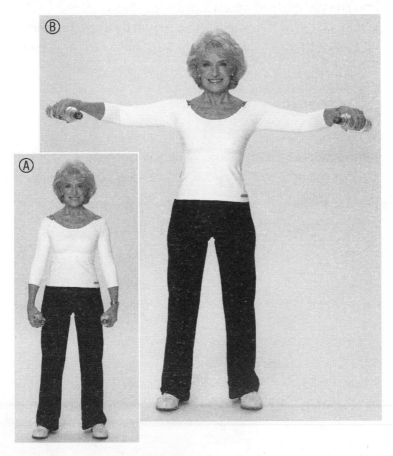

2 Waist shaper (2 × 8 reps each side)

Stand tall with your back straight and hold a handweight or water bottle in each hand, with the backs of your hands facing forward. Bring both arms in front at shoulder height Ⓐ. Now pull your left elbow back, bending the arm but keeping it at shoulder height, with shoulders down and relaxed Ⓑ. Keep watching the elbow

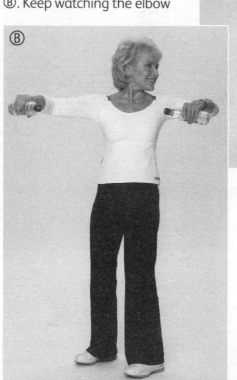

so your head turns as well and keep your hips facing front, with knees slightly bent. Do 8 reps to the same side, then change sides and repeat. Rest before doing another set.

3 Chest and underarm toner (2 × 12 reps)

Start on your hands and knees, with your hands under your shoulders and your knees under your hips, then move your knees further back and pull your tummy in Ⓐ. Breathe in as you lower your upper body towards the floor, bending your elbows outwards and leading with your chest Ⓑ. Breathe out as you push up again without locking your elbows. Do 12 reps, then rest and build up to another set.

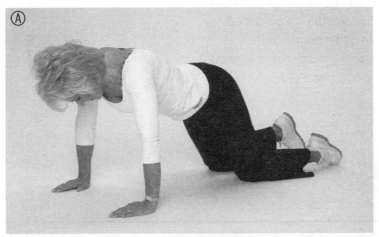

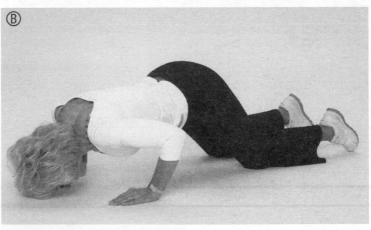

4 Tummy crunch (2 × 10 reps)

Lie on your back with legs raised and ankles crossed. Place both hands behind your head and pull your tummy in tight Ⓐ. Now breathe out as you lift your head and shoulders off the floor and, at the same time, lift your hips slightly Ⓑ. Keep your chin off your chest and hold your tummy in throughout. Do 10 reps, then rest before doing another set.

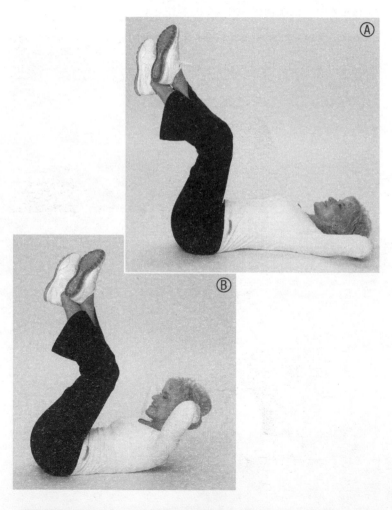

5 Advanced bottom shaper (2 × 8 reps alternate legs)
Lie on your back with knees bent, feet together and arms by
your sides Ⓐ. Now breathe in and, as you breathe out, lift your
hips off the floor without arching your back or coming up too
high and, at the same time, lift one leg to straighten it, keeping
your knees firmly together Ⓑ. Slowly lower your hips and leg,
then lift again and raise the other leg. Keep changing legs for
8 reps, then rest before doing another set.

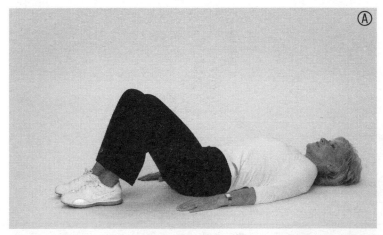

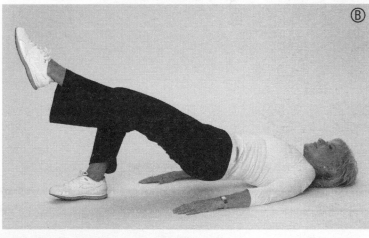

6 Advanced waist shaper (2 × 10 reps alternate sides)
Lie on your back with legs raised, ankles crossed and hands behind your head. Breathe out and as you lift your head and shoulders off the floor, reach one arm up and across towards the opposite foot. Lower again, then repeat to the other side. Keep changing sides for 10 reps, then rest before doing another set.

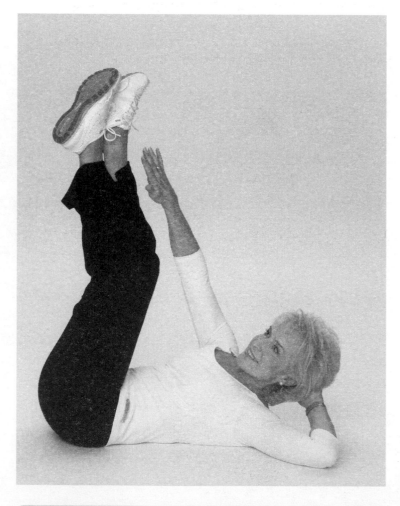

7 Outer thigh shaper with three-stage lift

(× 12 reps each leg)

Lie on your side and bend your bottom leg up to 90 degrees. Push the top leg out straight in line with your hip, with foot flexed, and hold a handweight or water bottle on the thigh. Pull your tummy in to hold your trunk still, then lift the top leg slightly and pause Ⓐ. Now lift the leg to mid range and pause again Ⓑ, then lift to the top of the range and pause Ⓒ, keeping your hips stacked. Lower under control in one movement, and repeat. Do 12 reps on one leg, then roll over and repeat the three-stage lift on the other leg.

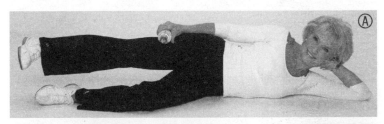

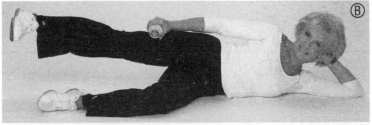

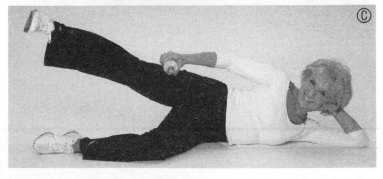

8 Inner thigh toner with two-stage lift

(× 16 reps each leg)

Lie on your side propped up on your elbow, with your top leg bent over the bottom leg and the knee resting on a rolled towel. Straighten the bottom leg and keep it off the floor slightly Ⓐ. Pull your tummy in to keep your trunk still and lift the bottom leg halfway up and pause Ⓑ. Now lift the leg to the top of the range Ⓒ before lowering again with a pause halfway down. Do 16 reps, then roll over, change legs and repeat.

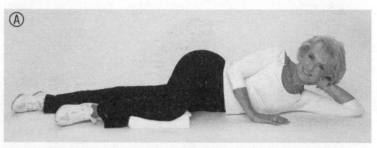

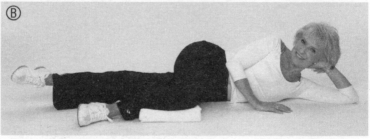

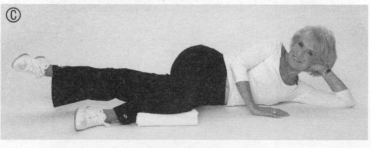

9 Full press-up (2 × 4 reps)

Come up onto your hands and knees and straighten your legs out behind, keeping your body in a straight line from the top of your head to your feet Ⓐ. Now breathe in and bend your elbows outwards, lowering your trunk to floor Ⓑ and holding your tummy in to support your back. Breathe out as you push up again. Do 4 reps, then rest before doing another set.

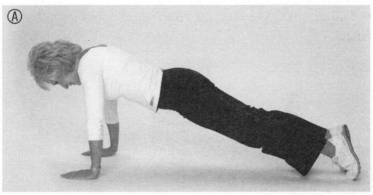

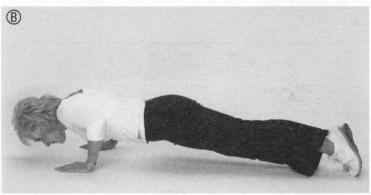

If a full press-up is too difficult, repeat Exercise 3 (chest and underarm toner) on p.279.

10 Posture improver and back strengthener (3 × 6 reps)
Lie on your front with your arms by your sides Ⓐ. Breathe out
as you pull your shoulders up and away from the floor Ⓑ, then
lift your head off floor but keep looking down, with your head
in line with your spine Ⓒ. Hold for 2 seconds, then breathe in
and lower slowly. Do 6 reps, then rest before doing 2 more sets.

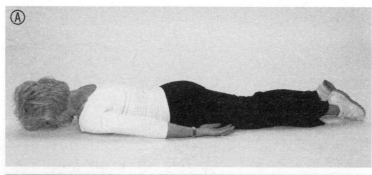

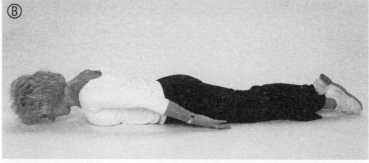

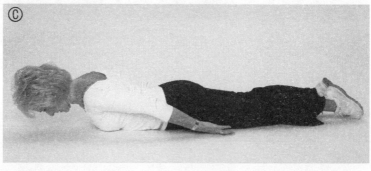

11 Tummy flattener ($\times$ 4 reps)

Lie on your front and come up onto your forearms and knees, with toes curled under. Now breathe in and, as you breathe out, pull your tummy in very tight and lift your knees off the floor so your body forms a straight line from the top of your head to your feet. Hold for 10 seconds, then release. Do 4 reps.

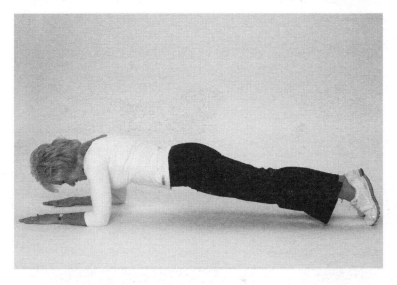

If you find this exercise too difficult, keep your knees on the floor.

Stretches

1 Tummy stretch

Lie on your front with your arms at your sides and your elbows bent. Keeping your hips in contact with the floor, prop up on your elbows and lift your chin forward slightly to feel a stretch in your tummy. Hold for 10 seconds, then release.

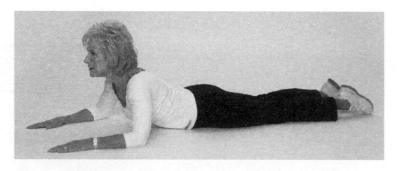

2 Back stretch

Come up onto your hands and knees and, as you pull your tummy in, arch your spine up towards the ceiling and let your head drop down. Hold for 10 seconds, then release.

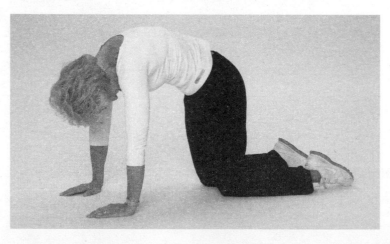

3 Waist stretch

Sit up tall with legs crossed, then lift your right arm and lean over to the left side, keeping both hips on floor and without leaning forward or back. Hold for 10 seconds, then release. Change sides and repeat.

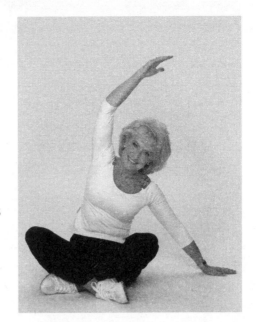

4 Chest stretch

Still sitting upright with legs crossed, place both hands behind you on the floor. Draw your shoulders back to feel a stretch across your chest and hold for 10 seconds, then release.

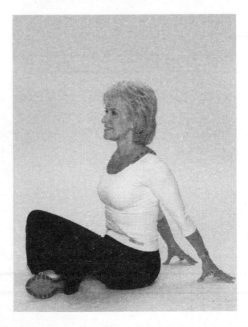

5 Underarm stretch

Place your right hand behind your right shoulder and use the pressure of your left hand on your right underarm to press the right hand further down your back. Keep your head up and look straight ahead. Hold for 10 seconds, then release. Change arms and repeat.

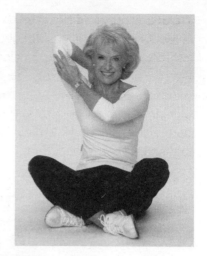

6 Back thigh stretch

Sit upright with one leg straight out in front and the other leg bent. Place your hands on the floor at either side of the straight leg and lean forwards from the hips to feel a stretch in back of the thigh. Hold for 10 seconds, then try to lean a little further forward for another 10 seconds. Change legs and repeat.

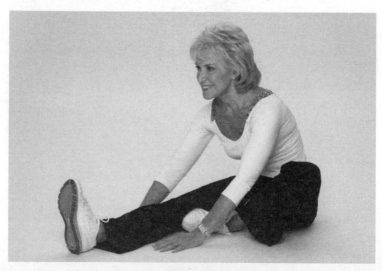

7 Outer thigh and hip stretch

Sit upright with your legs straight out in front and bring your left foot over the right leg, placing the foot flat on the floor. Place your left hand on the floor for support and your right hand across the left knee. Use the pressure of your right arm to pull the left leg further across your body to feel a stretch in the outer thigh and hip. Hold for 10 seconds, then release. Change legs and repeat.

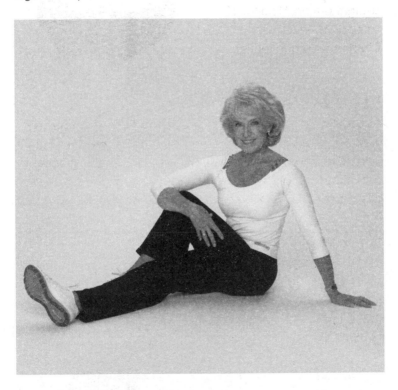

8 Inner thigh stretch

Sit upright with the soles of your feet together and your elbows resting on the insides of your thighs. Keeping your head up and your back straight, lean forwards and press your elbows onto your thighs. Hold for 10 seconds, then breathe in and, as you breathe out, press down further on your thighs and hold for another 10 seconds.

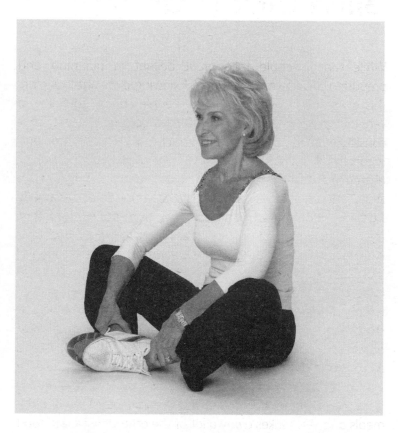

11 The Amazing Inch Loss Plan Solo Slim diet trial

While many people take great delight in planning and preparing their own meals when following a weight-loss plan, this doesn't suit everyone. Some people choose to follow a very-low-calorie diet of around 600–800 calories per day that consists mainly of the consumption of milkshakes and reconstituted powdery soups, because they find it easier to abstain from the temptations of normal food and they like the strict regimen of following a totally prescriptive diet. Personally I am not a fan of such 'unnatural' programmes as I feel that they do not re-educate the dieter to eat healthily and thus enable them to maintain their new weight in the future. For this reason, many dieters following a very-low-calorie diet regain part, if not all, of the weight they lose once they go back to eating normal food. However, I do understand that having a strict regime to follow is the only way that some people seem able to stick to a diet – rather like putting themselves in a 'food prison' for a few months!

My Amazing Inch Loss Plan Solo Slim diet is quite different from such regimes, because it offers proper, balanced healthy meals and yet it takes away a lot of the effort involved in food preparation. The diet plan is based on the same principles as the Amazing Inch Loss Plan diet (1200 calories for the first two weeks and 1400 calories for weeks three and four) but you order your chosen menu of meals online or by phone and have them delivered to your door in a Rosemary Conley Healthy Food Box, which comes with my low-fat Mature Cheese, Hot Chocolate Drinks and Low Gi Nutrition Bars. Once your food box arrives, you are all set to start the diet. All you have to do is add fruit, additional vegetables and your chosen breakfast menu to complete your week's menu. Individual SoloSlim® products are also available from Rosemary Conley Clubs.

The Solo Slim diet trial

To prove the effectiveness of the Amazing Inch Loss Plan Solo Slim diet I invited 30 volunteers to embark on a trial for one month. Unlike my previous diet trial, these folk were a mixture of new dieters and some who were already on their weight-loss journey but who had reached a bit of a plateau. I thought it would be interesting to see how they fared when given a fairly prescriptive eating plan with meals already prepared. The results were extremely encouraging and, between them, the 30 trialists lost a remarkable 32.2 stone in the month, making their average weight loss over four weeks an impressive 15lb. The biggest individual weight loss was 1st 9lb, and the lowest was 9lb. The Solo Slim diet works. It really, really works! Here are some of the comments from a few of the trialists.

Businesswoman Tricia Pedlar decided to lose weight and raise funds as part of an Executive Challenge in aid of charity and was thrilled when she lost 8lb in her first week. By the end of week four Tricia had lost 1st 2lb and was delighted. She said:

> I lead a busy life and found this is the only diet that really fitted in sensibly. I found the food very easy to stick to, delicious, and my kids and husband thought it smelled and tasted delicious too!

Robert Banner, who is the main organiser of the Executive Challenge, decided to raise funds for PROSTaid, a prostrate cancer charity based in Leicestershire, and volunteered to be a trialist on the Solo Slim Amazing Inch Loss Plan diet, and his wife, while not part of the trial, said she would join in as she needed to lose a little weight, too, and thought it would encourage Robert. Both are in their sixties. Robert only had a couple of stone to lose, and his wife was barely a stone overweight and it worried me slightly when she said that historically she found losing weight very difficult and could only shift a pound or two despite previous great efforts. She even admitted that she had 'been on diets for most of the last few years', so I was interested to see how she got along with Solo Slim. Robert lost a stone in the four weeks while his wife lost an impressive 9lb and was almost at her goal weight in a month! Robert said:

> The weight was dropping off before I knew it! Your diet really works and gives the results that it promises.

I also had a mother and two-daughter team on the trial. Mum Elspeth Williamson-Carr lost a remarkable 1st 5lb in the month. Daughter Abigail lost 1st 2lb and Amymay lost 10lb. Their inch losses were impressive, too, as they lost 17 inches, 12 inches and 10 inches respectively in the four weeks. Elspeth commented:

> This has been a life-changing experience. This is the easiest, healthiest way to lose weight. The food is lovely and tasty and I would say to anyone, if it can work for me it can work for you!

Daughter Abigail said:

> I was very shocked at my final weigh-in when I was told that I had lost 1st 2lb over the four-week trial. I

am thrilled to bits with this result and feel that it has given me a huge kick-start into getting back into shape. I would recommend this diet to anyone as it is very easy to follow and the meals are like home-cooked food, not like other diets that are shakes/drink-based. If anything, on this diet you struggle to eat all the food you can in a day so you never feel hungry and therefore you don't crave food. It's a fantastic start to getting back on track.

Fifty-seven-year-old Maureen Squires, from Leeds, lost 1st 1lb during the four-week trial and reduced her BMI from an unhealthy 27.3 to a healthy 25, which is terrific. She wrote:

Just a huge thank you! This has been the one diet that has worked for me. I found it so much easier to follow with the meals and menu sorted out for you. I am two sizes smaller and in trousers I have not worn for years! I feel much healthier and am enjoying walking. As I have had two hip replacements, the benefits are fantastic. The joints feel great!

As well as our weekly classes at Rosemary Conley Diet and Fitness Clubs, we also run an online slimming club, www.rosemaryconleyonline.com. One of my Solo Slim trialists was an online member who wishes to stay anonymous. She wrote:

After an initial great start on rosemaryconleyonline, I faltered. Doing the four-week trial really helped me regain my focus and I was thrilled to lose 13.2lb and 20 inches in four weeks – especially as this period included many social events. For me, the set nature of the diet really helped me to stick to it, as I wasn't distracted by lots of other choices – it made it very clear-cut.

Mavis Smith is in her mid-sixties and attends our classes in Norfolk. Despite having already lost a stone, Mavis lost 10lb on the Solo Slim trial. She wrote:

*When on previous diets, I had just given in to really bad cravings. To feel in control of them is really great and I now feel maybe I **will** be slim – forget the maybe! It's been wonderful not to have to think 'what shall we eat tonight?' For two weeks of the four we've had our family staying and it's been so easy getting their meals and just heating up my own!*

Jean Winslett, who's 73, wrote:

In all my many years of dieting I have never found an easier way of losing weight. Although I didn't quite make a stone (I lost 13lb), it has given me the incentive to press on and reach my personal goal of 1½ stone. I have really enjoyed exercising every day using a combination of three-mile brisk walking and two or three weekly visits to the gym for toning, and I will certainly be keeping this going and I feel energised by it.

Isn't that brilliant? Well done, Jean!

Husband and wife team, Julie and Tony Wells, decided to do the diet together. Julie wasn't very overweight at 10st 7lb for her 5ft 3in height and a BMI of 26.1 at the start of the trial, while Tony, who is 5ft 11in tall, weighed in at 14st 6lb.

Julie wrote:

We started this diet just before we went on a three-week holiday on a canal boat. The Solo Slim food was easy to store as it didn't need refrigerating. I found the Power Snacks very useful as around mid-morning, after taking the boat through many locks, we needed a little treat. This is the first time I have been on holiday and lost weight at the same time!

After four weeks Julie had lost 11lb and now has a healthy BMI of 24.2. Tony had lost an astonishing 1st 9lb, and his BMI fell from 28.2 to 25 in the month. To drop from 14st 6lb to 12st 11lb in just four weeks is an incredible achievement.

Tony commented:

I found the diet easy to follow and I feel fitter, have a great deal more energy, and my overall health has improved tremendously. Thank you!

Another husband and wife team were Kevin and Karen Chapman. Kevin, 56, lost 1st 5lb and 24 inches in the month's trial, while his wife Karen lost 10lb and 12 inches. Kevin said:

This is the most weight I have ever lost on any diet and, with Karen and I slimming together and eating the ready meals, it has made it so much easier. We can have different menus to suit our personal taste without any bother. Solo Slim is just so easy!

I also recruited some trialists from my own classes that I run on Monday evenings. When Laura and Karen joined in August 2010, I asked if they would like to participate, and they were delighted to accept the challenge. In week one Karen lost 8lb and Laura lost 7lb! Week two saw Laura leap ahead with a further 5lb loss, making a total loss of 12lb in just two weeks. Karen lost 2lb in week two, making a total loss of 10lb in 14 days, which was very impressive.

By the end of four weeks Karen had lost 13lb and 14 inches, and Laura had lost 1st 1lb and a total of 13 inches, so they were both very happy with their results.

Karen wrote:

Not only has the trial made me look at my eating habits, it has also made me re-evaluate my lifestyle. Now I find going to the gym rewarding, rather than punishing. I realise the benefits of healthy eating, along with exercise, and I have a positive outlook on my weight-loss goal. Rather than looking at my goal as impossible, the trial has given me the motivation and the boost to realise that it's totally possible, and in fact I can't wait for the challenge!

Laura wrote:

The Solo Slim diet is the easiest diet I have ever followed and I didn't feel hungry like I have with other diets. With so many different and delicious meals to choose from, it doesn't feel like I'm dieting at all. I have tried low-fat cheese before but it just doesn't taste the same. The Rosemary Conley cheese is different – full of flavour and it tastes great! My favourite meal is the Thai chicken. It's the meal I saved for when I wanted a treat! Far better than the full-fat versions I've had before. I feel healthier now than I have in years!

When Julie Bamford joined my class in April 2010 she was determined to sort out her weight. Diagnosed with a thyroid problem, but now taking the appropriate medication, Julie had found herself morbidly obese and desperate to lose weight. In three months, she managed to shed an impressive 2st 11lb, but then her weight loss slowed down and she was getting impatient. When I offered her the chance to become a trialist for Solo Slim, she was delighted. In her first week she lost 6lb, then another 4lb in week two. The third week it was 2lb and in week four she lost another 5lb. In total Julie lost 1st 3lb in the month and was well on her way to losing her fourth stone in four months. Julie is so motivated by what Solo Slim has done for her. She said:

I know I'm impatient, but I was getting frustrated when the weight loss slowed down. The Solo Slim trial has kick-started my weight loss and motivated me to do more exercise. For people who struggle with choices of healthy food, Solo Slim is ideal. I feel energetic and alive. I walk further than ever before and my dog loves the new me! I take the stairs at every work setting I visit and haven't used the lifts in four months.

It was a very exciting moment two weeks later when I presented Julie with her 'four stone certificate' at my class. She looks a totally different person now.

Gabi Tarjanyi has been attending my class on and off since 2003. Over that time she has lost about 1 stone, but sometimes a few pounds creep back on and she works hard to try to lose them again. Gabi comes to class with her friend, Carole, who has a similar track record of progress, apart from when her son got married and she lost a couple of stone for the wedding. Gabi and Carole are typical middle-aged ladies who have been dieting for most of their adult lives and, although they have very good intentions, life often gets in the way. So when they approached me and asked 'please can we be trial dieters for Solo Slim?', I was unsure at first. I needed my trialists to be totally dedicated and I wasn't convinced that they could deliver. Nevertheless, I agreed. If Solo Slim worked for Gabi and Carole, it could work for anyone. This would be a real test, I thought.

At the first weigh-in Gabi had lost 6lb! The next week it was another 1½lb off and by the end of four weeks, Gabby had lost an amazing 12lb!

This is what she said:

> I've been struggling and yo-yo dieting for years but the Solo Slim diet plan was so easy to follow, with no preparing meals from scratch, that I have achieved a fantastic 12lb weight loss in four weeks – I am so happy! The kick-start that Solo Slim has given me has made me more determined than ever to continue with my weight loss. I also feel re-educated about my diet and portion sizes.

Carole, meanwhile, lost 4lb in week one and was thrilled. By the end of week two another couple of pounds had disappeared – that was almost half a stone in two weeks – and by the end of the month she had lost a total of 10lb. Carole was thrilled and both she and Gabi decided that they were going to carry on with the Solo Slim food boxes as it really worked for them. One comment from Carole said it all:

> It has really made me realise where I've been going wrong. It's portion size, and yet when I eat the Solo

Slim meals I realise that I've had enough and that I really don't need more! It's been life-changing for me!

As you can see, the Amazing Inch Loss Plan Solo Slim diet worked brilliantly for our trial dieters and it can work just as well for you. The benefits are that, with the excellent range of menus available, you should never get bored, and having the meals delivered directly to your door really does make life easier. The Solo Slim meals are easy to prepare and extremely satisfying. I eat them myself, as does my husband Mike, and we both find them delicious. The staff at our offices love eating them for lunch, and I know that you'll love them too.

So, whether you want to give your diet a big boost, or build Solo Slim into your everyday life or follow it on just a couple of days a week when you reach your goal weight, Solo Slim is there to help you. You don't have to commit to buying a month's worth of food; just buy it when you want. You can buy it by mail order through www.rosemaryconley.com or buy individual meals at our classes, along with my low-fat Mature Cheese (5% fat) and Low Gi Nutrition Bars and Solo Slim® Hot Chocolate Drinks.

My low-fat cheese is, without doubt, the best low-fat cheese on the market. We are able to send it in the post because it is a mature cheese and we can deliver it within 24 hours. The cheese is made using the highest-quality milk from extremely well-cared for cows. I have been to Wyke Farms, where the cheese is made, and met the cows from which the cheese is created! You can log on to www.rosemaryconley.tv and meet them too!

My Low Gi Nutrition Bars come in three flavours – Peach and Raspberry, Apple and Cinnamon, and Ginger. They are made from high-quality natural products (and are not to be confused with cereal bars, which are significantly more processed). They will keep you feeling full for hours. Just half a bar makes the perfect Power Snack to get you through the morning or afternoon until your next meal time. Alternatively, you can use them as part of a breakfast or lunch. I recommend you take them with a drink to help you fill up even more.

My Solo Slim® Hot Chocolate Drinks come in two flavours – Chocolate, and Chocolate and Orange. Just make them up with water in a cup or, for a really luxuriously creamy drink, make them up with milk from your daily allowance.

We will keep adding more meal choices to the Solo Slim® range, so check out the website for the latest additions. By the time you buy this book the range will have grown, so you will be able to substitute different evening meals for the ones listed in the next chapter – just check the calories on each pack (these details are on the website).

I hope you enjoy the Amazing Inch Loss Plan Solo Slim diet and I look forward to hearing from you about your remarkable results.

12 The Amazing Inch Loss Plan Solo Slim diet and meal planner

As each individual's food preferences, tastes and lifestyle habits vary, I have simply listed lots of menu options for breakfast, lunch and dinner, rather than giving a day-to-day menu plan, although I have included an example of what a week's menu might look like.

All the breakfasts are based on 200 calories, all the lunches on 300 calories and all the dinners on 400 calories. It's important for you to have your 450ml (¾ pint) of milk each day in addition to your three meals and your two 50-calorie Power Snacks. The Power Snacks can be combined to make one larger snack if that suits you better. After two weeks you can add 200 calories a day in the form of 1 alcoholic drink or 1 high-fat treat and 1 low-fat dessert (max. 100 kcal each).

Don't forget to check www.rosemaryconley.com for details of new meals and products in the Solo Slim® range. Just check the calories, which are included on the website, and make your own substitutions if you like.

Maximising your weight and inch loss

As with the Amazing Inch Loss Plan elsewhere in this book it is important to combine your Solo Slim diet with regular exercise and physical activity. Follow the daily aerobic challenges on pages 92–203 and combine this with the daily toning exercises by logging on to www.rosemaryconley.tv/ailpDay1, ailpDay2, etc. If you don't have access to a computer, then the exercise programme is available in my original Amazing Inch Loss Plan book, which you can order by calling our mail order number on 0870 0507727. Follow the exercises in the sequence given as they are progressive in both intensity and duration.

If you stick strictly to 1200 calories a day for the first two weeks (14-Day Fast Track) and then 1400 calories a day for weeks three and four (14-Day 1400) and do the recommended exercises, I guarantee that you will lose weight and inches. At the end of week four turn to pages 378–9 to find your new personal calorie allowance, which is determined by your age, gender and weight, so that you can continue to lose weight. As you lose each further half stone, adjust your calorie allowance accordingly by checking against the appropriate column on the chart. After you've reached your ideal weight, then obviously you can be more relaxed. Please see pages 374–6 for advice and help with maintaining your weight loss in the long term.

The Amazing Inch Loss Plan Solo Slim diet

Daily allowance

Weeks 1 and 2: 14-Day Fast Track

Breakfast	200 kcal
Mid-morning Power Snack	50 kcal
Lunch	300 kcal
Mid-afternoon Power Snack	50 kcal
Dinner	400 kcal
450ml (¾ pint) skimmed or semi-skimmed milk	200 kcal
Total (Weeks 1 and 2)	**1200 kcal**

During this two-week period avoid alcohol or any extras.

Add-ons for Weeks 3 and 4: 14-Day 1400

1 alcoholic drink *or* 1 high-fat treat	100 kcal
1 low-fat dessert	100 kcal
Total (Weeks 3 and 4)	**1400 kcal**

If you have any special dietary requirements, then our mail order department (telephone 0870 0507727) will be happy to help you select your meals. Providing your order is received by 12 noon, from Monday to Thursday, you can be assured that delivery will take place within 24 hours. Your week's supply will come in a smart Rosemary Conley Healthy Food Box, which makes a very nice storage box for you to use at home in the future.

The 7-day Solo Slim diet

This sample 7-day Solo Slim diet is based on 1200 calories per day. Don't forget to include your daily milk allowance of 450ml (¾ pint) skimmed or semi-skimmed milk. After the initial two weeks and if your calorie allowance permits, you can add in an alcoholic drink or high-fat treat and a low-fat dessert (max. 100 kcal each).

DAY 1

Breakfast (200 kcal)
■ 1 × **Rosemary Conley Low Gi Nutrition Bar** (any flavour) plus 2 pieces fresh fruit of your choice (excluding bananas) ☑

Mid-morning power snack (50 kcal)
■ 1 × **Rosemary Conley Solo Slim®Hot Chocolate Drink** made in a cup of water or with milk from allowance

Lunch (300 kcal)
■ 1 × **Solo Slim® Low-Fat Carrot and Coriander Soup** served with a small wholegrain bread roll, followed by 100g fresh fruit salad ☑

Mid-afternoon power snack (50 kcal)
■ 1 satsuma and 1 kiwi fruit ☑

Dinner (400 kcal)
■ 1 × **Solo Slim® Low-Fat Chicken Hotpot** served with 100g broccoli and 100g cabbage or carrots, followed by 1 low-fat yogurt (max. 100 kcal and 5% fat)

DAY 2

Breakfast (200 kcal)
- 2 Weetabix or Shredded Wheat served with milk from allowance plus 1 tsp sugar ☑

Mid-morning power snack (50 kcal)
- 1 fresh pear or mini banana ☑

Lunch (300 kcal)
- 1 × **Solo Slim® Low-Fat Spicy Beef and Tomato Soup** served with 2 Ryvitas spread with 1 tsp very-low-fat mayonnaise and topped with 25g grated **Rosemary Conley low-fat Mature Cheese** and 1 sliced tomato

Mid-afternoon power snack (50 kcal)
- 1 small apple or orange ☑

Dinner (400 kcal)
- 1 × **Solo Slim® Low-Fat Mushroom Soup** plus 1 × **Solo Slim® Low-Fat Chilli and Rice**

> Rosemary Conley Solo Slim® meals and soups can be heated in the microwave, in a saucepan on the hob or in a casserole in the oven.

DAY 3

Breakfast (200 kcal)
▪ ½ fresh grapefruit plus 1 medium-sized egg, boiled or poached, served with 1 slice wholegrain bread, toasted and spread with Marmite ☑

Mid-morning power snack (50 kcal)
▪ 1 × **Rosemary Conley Solo Slim® Hot Chocolate Drink** made in a cup with water or with milk from allowance

Lunch (300 kcal)
▪ 1 × **Solo Slim® Low-Fat Lentil Soup** served with a large salad and 100g chicken/beef/ham or 40g **Rosemary Conley low-fat Mature Cheese** plus 1 tsp very-low-fat mayonnaise ☑

Mid-afternoon power snack (50 kcal)
▪ Chop up 1 peeled carrot, 2 sticks celery and 1 × 5cm piece cucumber and serve with a dip made with 1 tsp very-low-fat mayonnaise and a pinch of chilli powder ☑

Dinner (400 kcal)
▪ 1 × **Solo Slim® Low-Fat Tomato and Vegetable Pasta** served with small salad tossed in fat-free dressing, followed by 100g fresh fruit salad topped with 1 tsp Total 0% fat Greek Yoghurt ☑

DAY 4

Breakfast (200 kcal)
▓ 1 × 100g pot low-fat natural yogurt (max. 75 kcal and 5 % fat) mixed with 1 tbsp unsweetened muesli and 1 red Portion Pot® (115g) fresh raspberries ☑

Mid-morning power snack (50 kcal)
▓ ½ × **Rosemary Conley Low Gi Nutrition Bar** ☑

Lunch (300 kcal)
▓ 2 slices wholegrain bread spread with very-low-fat mayonnaise made into a sandwich with 25g grated **Rosemary Conley low-fat Mature Cheese**, 1 large sliced tomato, salad leaves, 1 sliced red onion and 4 slices cucumber ☑

Mid-afternoon power snack (50 kcal)
▓ ½ × **Rosemary Conley Low Gi Nutrition Bar** ☑

Dinner (400 kcal)
▓ 1 × **Solo Slim® Low-Fat Tomato Soup** plus 1 × **Solo Slim® Low-Fat Beef Casserole** served with 100g broccoli or cabbage

DAY 5

Breakfast (200 kcal)
▓ 1 yellow Portion Pot® (125ml) fresh orange juice plus 1 red Portion Pot® (40g) Special K cereal served with milk from allowance and 1 tsp sugar ☑

Mid-morning power snack (50 kcal)
▓ 1 Ryvita spread with Marmite and topped with a large sliced tomato ☑

Lunch (300 kcal)
▓ 1 slice wholegrain bread, toasted, with 30g Rosemary Conley low-fat Mature Cheese and a dash of Worcestershire sauce, followed by 1 × **Rosemary Conley Low Gi Nutrition Bar** and 1 small pear ☑

Mid-afternoon power snack (50 kcal)
▓ 2 satsumas or 2 kiwi fruits ☑

Dinner (400 kcal)
▓ 1 × **Solo Slim® Low-Fat Lamb Hotpot** served with 100g boiled new potatoes (with skins) and 100g green vegetables of your choice

DAY 6

Breakfast (200 kcal)
- 1 slice toasted wholegrain toast topped with 1 yellow Portion Pot® (115g) baked beans, followed by 1 piece fresh fruit ☑

Mid-morning power snack (50 kcal)
- 75g seedless grapes ☑

Lunch (300 kcal)
- 1 × **Solo Slim® Low-Fat Pea and Ham Soup** plus 1 slice wholegrain bread, toasted, with 30g Rosemary Conley low-fat Mature Cheese and a dash of Worcestershire sauce served with a large salad tossed in fat-free dressing ☑

Mid-afternoon power snack (50 kcal)
- 1 fresh peach or 150g strawberries ☑

Dinner (400 kcal)
- 1 × **Solo Slim® Low-Fat Thai Chicken Curry** served with 25g (dry weight) basmati rice, boiled in water with a vegetable stock cube

DAY 7

Breakfast (200 kcal)
▓ 1 small banana, sliced, mixed with 115g sliced strawberries and 1 × 100g pot yogurt (max. 100 kcal and 5% fat) ☑

Mid-morning power snack (50 kcal)
▓ 20g sultanas ☑

Lunch (300 kcal)
▓ 2 slices wholegrain bread spread with very-low-fat cream cheese (e.g. Philadelphia Extra Light) and topped with 30g smoked salmon served with a small rocket salad

Mid-afternoon power snack (50 kcal)
▓ 100g fresh pineapple ☑

Dinner (400 kcal)
▓ 1 × **Solo Slim® Low-Fat Three Bean and Chorizo Soup** plus 1 × **Solo Slim® Low-Fat Beef Casserole** served with 100g green vegetables of your choice

---

This 7-day menu is based on a sample Rosemary Conley Health Food Box and comprises 7 soups, 7 ready meals, a pack of Low Gi Nutrition Bars and a pack of Rosemary Conley low-fat Mature Cheese.

The Solo Slim meal planner

Daily allowance

**Weeks 1 and 2
14-Day Fast Track**

Breakfast	200 kcal
Mid-morning Power Snack	50 kcal
Lunch	300 kcal
Mid-afternoon Power Snack	50 kcal
Dinner	400 kcal
450ml (¾ pint) skimmed or semi-skimmed milk	200 kcal
Total (Weeks 1 and 2)	**1200 kcal**

During this two-week period avoid alcohol or any extras.

**Add-ons for Weeks 3 and 4
14-Day 1400**

1 alcoholic drink *or* 1 high-fat treat	100 kcal
1 low-fat dessert	100 kcal
Total (Weeks 3 and 4)	**1400 kcal**

> Remember to do the daily aerobic fitness challenges to achieve maximum weight and inch loss (see p.338).

BREAKFASTS

Approx. 200 kcal each; choose one per day

Cereal breakfasts

▩ 1 green Portion Pot® (50g) Special K cereal plus milk from allowance and 1 tsp sugar ☑

▩ 1 yellow Portion Pot® (30g) fruit and fibre cereal served with milk from allowance and topped with 1 red Portion Pot® (115g) fresh raspberries or 1 tsp sugar ☑

▩ 1 red Portion Pot® (50g) fruit and fibre cereal (or any bran cereal), served with milk from allowance and 10 seedless grapes ☑

▩ 1 Weetabix or Shredded Wheat served with milk from allowance plus 1 tsp sugar and 1 thinly sliced medium banana ☑

▩ 2 Weetabix served with milk from allowance and 2 tsps sugar or 1 mini banana ☑

▩ 1 yellow Portion Pot® (14 Minis) Weetabix Fruit 'n' Nut Minis, plus 1 medium banana, sliced, served with milk from allowance ☑

▩ 1 yellow Portion Pot® (30g) All-Bran served with milk from allowance and 1 tsp sugar, plus 1 boiled egg ☑

▩ 1 red Portion Pot® (30g) Sugar Puffs mixed with 115g canned peaches in natural juice ☑

▩ Mix 100g 0% fat Greek yogurt with 1 blue Portion Pot® (40g) muesli and a little semi-skimmed milk from allowance to moisten. Add a little Silver Spoon Half Spoon to sweeten to taste. Leave to soak overnight in the refrigerator for best results. Serve chilled ☑

▩ 1 blue Portion Pot® (35g) uncooked porridge oats, cooked in water with 10 sultanas and served with milk from allowance ☑

Fruit breakfasts

■ 1 Müllerlight yogurt, any flavour (max. 150 kcal), plus 1 small banana
■ 2 large bananas ☑
■ Frozen Berry Smoothie (see recipe, p.272) ☑
■ Fruit Smoothie: blend 150g fresh fruit (peaches, strawberries, raspberries or blueberries) with 100g Total 2% fat Greek Yoghurt and milk from allowance ☑
■ 1 small banana, sliced, mixed with 115g sliced strawberries and 1 × 100g pot low-fat yogurt, any flavour (max. 100 kcal and 5% fat) ☑
■ 200g fresh fruit salad topped with 100g Total 2% fat Greek Yoghurt and 6 sultanas ☑
■ 100g Total 2% fat Greek Yoghurt mixed with 140g fresh fruit, sweetened to taste with a little Silver Spoon Half Spoon ☑

Quick and easy breakfasts

■ 1 yellow Portion Pot® (125ml) fresh orange juice, plus 1 slice wholegrain bread spread with 2 tsps marmalade, jam or honey ☑
■ ½ fresh grapefruit plus 2 boiled medium-sized eggs ☑ℙ
■ ½ bagel (or 1 whole mini bagel) toasted, spread with 1 tsp fruit preserve, jam, honey or marmalade, then topped with 50g Total 2% fat Greek Yoghurt ☑
■ 200g Total 2% fat Greek Yoghurt mixed with 1 tsp runny honey ☑
■ 4 prunes, soaked overnight in 1 blue Portion Pot® (80g) low-fat natural yogurt, mixed with 1 tsp porridge oats ☑

Cooked breakfasts

■ 2 well-grilled back bacon rashers or 2 Quorn sausages, grilled, served with 1 dry-fried medium-sized egg, 3 tomatoes, halved and grilled, and 5 grilled mushrooms ☑ℙ

■ 2 low-fat (max. 5% fat) beef, pork or Quorn sausages, grilled, served with 1 yellow Portion Pot® (115g) baked beans and 50g grilled mushrooms ☑️P

■ 2 Quorn sausages, grilled, served with 1 dry-fried medium-sized egg and 1 × 200g can tomatoes, boiled until reduced ☑️P

■ 2 Quorn sausages, grilled, served with 1 × 400g can tomatoes boiled until reduced, plus 50g grilled mushrooms ☑️P

■ 1 Quorn Bacon Style Rasher, grilled, served with 1 yellow Portion Pot® (115g) baked beans plus 1 tomato, halved and grilled, and 50g grilled mushrooms ☑️P

■ Tomatoes and Mushrooms on Toast: Boil 1 × 400g can chopped tomatoes well to reduce to a thick consistency and season well with freshly ground black pepper. Spoon onto 1 toasted large slice wholegrain bread and serve with 10 grilled mushrooms ☑️

■ ½ fresh grapefruit plus 1 poached medium-sized egg served on 1 toasted small slice wholegrain bread spread with Marmite ☑️

■ 2 eggs scrambled with milk from allowance and served with 100g grilled tomatoes and unlimited grilled mushrooms ☑️P

■ 2-egg omelette made using milk from allowance, dry-fried and filled with chopped mushrooms, sliced cherry tomatoes and freshly ground black pepper ☑️

■ 2 turkey rashers and 1 low-fat beef or pork sausage (max. 5% fat), grilled or dry-fried, served with 1 × 200g can tomatoes boiled until reduced and 100g grilled mushrooms P

■ 4 turkey rashers, grilled, served with 100g grilled, sliced mushrooms and 2 large tomatoes, grilled ☑️P

■ 4 turkey rashers, grilled, served with 1 dry-fried medium-sized egg, 1 × 200g can plum tomatoes, boiled until reduced, and 5 grilled mushrooms P

■ 2 turkey rashers, grilled, served with 1 yellow Portion Pot® (115g) baked beans and 1 dry-fried medium-sized egg **P**

■ 1 slice wholegrain bread, toasted, topped with 1 yellow Portion Pot® (115g) baked beans ✓

■ 1 slice wholegrain bread, soaked in 1 beaten egg and milk from allowance, fried in a little spray oil and topped with 1 tsp maple syrup ✓

■ 1 small slice multigrain bread, toasted, served with 1 egg, scrambled, boiled or dry-fried; plus ½ pink grapefruit ✓

■ 1 slice wholegrain bread, toasted, spread with savoury sauce (e.g. tomato ketchup, brown sauce or fruity sauce), then topped with 2 grilled turkey rashers plus 3 grilled tomatoes

■ 1 slice wholegrain bread, toasted, topped with 1 scrambled egg and 2 grilled tomatoes ✓

■ 1 blue Portion Pot® (35g) uncooked porridge oats, cooked in water with 10 sultanas and served with milk from allowance ✓

LUNCHES

Approx. 300 kcal each; choose one per day

Non-vegetarian lunches

■ 1 × **Solo Slim® Low-Fat Three Bean and Chorizo Soup** served with 1 medium slice wholegrain bread, toasted, topped with 25g **Rosemary Conley low-fat Mature Cheese**

■ 1 × **Solo Slim® Low-Fat Three Bean and Chorizo Soup** plus a small salad served with 40g wafer thin ham/beef/chicken/turkey and fat-free salad dressing

■ 1 × **Solo Slim® Low-Fat Three Bean and Chorizo Soup**, followed by 1 low-fat yogurt (max. 140 kcal and 5% fat)

■ 1 × **Solo Slim® Low-Fat Lentil Soup** plus a large salad and 75g chicken (no skin) or 100g ham served with 30g very-low-fat mayonnaise

▓ 1 × **Solo Slim® Low-Fat Pea and Ham Soup** plus 1 slice wholegrain bread spread with 1 tsp very-low-fat mayonnaise and topped with salad leaves, sliced tomatoes and 25g grated **Rosemary Conley low-fat Mature Cheese**

▓ 1 × **Solo Slim® Low-Fat Carrot and Coriander Soup** plus an open sandwich made with 1 medium slice wholegrain bread spread with 20g very-low-fat mayonnaise and topped with 100g wafer thin ham and salad

▓ 1 × **Solo Slim® Low-Fat Carrot and Coriander Soup** plus 1 × 6-pack Morrison's Eat Smart Melba Toast spread with 2 × Laughing Cow Extra Light Cheese Triangles, followed by 1 × **Rosemary Conley Low Gi Nutrition Bar**

▓ 1 × **Solo Slim® Low-Fat Carrot and Coriander Soup** plus 1 pack Splendips Sweet Chilli Flavour, followed by 1 × Hartley's Low Calorie Jelly (any flavour) served with 60g low-fat yogurt

▓ 1 × **Solo Slim® Low-Fat Spicy Beef and Tomato Soup** served with 1 medium slice wholegrain bread

▓ 1 × **Solo Slim® Low-Fat Spicy Beef and Tomato Soup**, followed by 1 low-fat yogurt (max. 135 kcal and 5% fat)

▓ 1 × **Solo Slim® Low-Fat Spicy Beef and Tomato Soup** plus 2 Ryvitas spread with extra light soft cheese

▓ 1 × **Solo Slim® Low-Fat Spicy Beef and Tomato Soup** served with 60g vegetable crudités and 100g mint and yogurt dip, followed by 1 fresh pear

▓ **1 × Solo Slim® Low-Fat Spicy Beef and Tomato Soup** served with 2 ready-to-eat poppadoms, followed by 150g strawberries

▓ 1 × **Solo Slim® Low-Fat Spicy Beef and Tomato Soup** served with 1 small wholemeal pitta bread

▓ 1 × **Solo Slim® Low-Fat Pea and Ham Soup** plus 1 slice wholegrain bread, toasted, topped with 30g **Rosemary Conley low-fat Mature Cheese** and dash of Worcestershire sauce

- 1 × **Solo Slim® Low-Fat Carrot and Coriander Soup** plus 1 × **Solo Slim® Low-Fat Three Bean Casserole**, followed by 1 × Hartley's Low Calorie Jelly, any flavour
- 1 × **Solo Slim® Low-Fat Pea and Ham Soup** plus a small salad topped with 50g grated **Rosemary Conley low-fat Mature Cheese** and 1 tsp very-low-fat mayonnaise
- 1 × **Solo Slim® Low-Fat Tomato Soup**, followed by 1 × Müllerlight yogurt (max. 120 kcal and 5% fat) and 75g strawberries
- 1 × **Solo Slim® Low-Fat Thai Chicken Curry**
- 1 × **Solo Slim® Low-Fat Chilli and Rice**
- 1 × **Solo Slim® Low-Fat Beef Casserole**, followed by 1 large banana and 1 kiwi fruit
- 1 × **Solo Slim® Low-Fat Beef Casserole**, followed by 1 low-fat yogurt (max. 125 kcal and 5% fat)
- 1 × **Solo Slim® Low-Fat Beef Casserole** served with a mixed salad tossed in fat-free dressing
- 1 × **Solo Slim® Low-Fat Mushroom Soup**, followed by 1 × **Solo Slim® Low-Fat Beef Casserole**
- 1 × **Solo Slim® Low-Fat Beef Meatballs and Potato**
- 1 × **Solo Slim® Low-Fat Lamb Hotpot**, followed by 1 kiwi fruit or satsuma
- 1 × **Solo Slim® Low-Fat Chicken Hotpot**, followed by 1 kiwi fruit or satsuma
- 1 × **Solo Slim® Low-Fat Tomato Soup** served with a small mixed salad and 50g wafer thin ham/turkey/chicken/beef and very-low-fat dressing
- 1 × **Solo Slim® Low-Fat Minestrone Soup** plus 1 × **Solo Slim® Low-Fat Beef Casserole**

Vegetarian lunches
- 1 × **Solo Slim® Low-Fat Lentil Soup** served with 1 small wholegrain bread roll (max. 100 kcal), followed by 1 apple ☑

- 1 × **Solo Slim® Low-Fat Lentil Soup** served with a large salad and 50g grated **Rosemary Conley low-fat Mature Cheese** plus 30g very-low-fat mayonnaise ✓
- 1 × **Solo Slim® Low-Fat Lentil Soup**, followed by 1 × **Rosemary Conley Low Gi Nutrition Bar** and 1 × **Rosemary Conley Solo Slim® Hot Chocolate Drink** made in a cup with water or with milk from allowance ✓
- 1 × **Solo Slim® Low-Fat Carrot and Coriander Soup** served with 1 small wholegrain bread roll (max. 100 kcal), followed by 100g fresh fruit salad made up of 30g grapes, 30g oranges, 20g apples and 20g pineapple ✓
- 1 × **Solo Slim® Low-Fat Carrot and Coriander Soup**, followed by 1 × **Rosemary Conley Low Gi Nutrition Bar**, plus 1 small banana ✓
- 1 × **Solo Slim® Low-Fat Minestrone Soup**, followed by 1 × **Rosemary Conley Low Gi Nutrition Bar** and 1 medium banana ✓
- 1 × **Solo Slim® Low-Fat Minestrone Soup** plus a small salad served with 50g low-fat cottage cheese topped with 25g grated **Rosemary Conley low-fat Mature Cheese** and 1 tsp very-low-fat mayonnaise ✓
- 1 × **Solo Slim® Low-Fat Three Bean Casserole** followed by 1 × **Rosemary Conley Low Gi Nutrition Bar** ✓
- 1 × **Solo Slim® Low-Fat Spicy Vegetable and Lentil Dahl**, followed by 1 low-fat yogurt (max. 60 kcal and 5% fat) ✓
- 1 × **Solo Slim® Low-Fat Tomato and Vegetable Pasta**, followed by 1 apple and 1 satsuma ✓
- 1 × **Solo Slim® Low-Fat Tomato and Vegetable Pasta**, followed by 1 medium banana ✓
- 1 × **Solo Slim® Low-Fat Mushroom Soup** plus a 2-egg omelette made using milk from allowance and filled with 25g grated **Rosemary Conley low-fat Mature Cheese** and sliced cherry tomatoes ✓

■ 1 × **Solo Slim® Low-Fat Tomato and Vegetable Pasta** served with a small salad and 25g grated **Rosemary Conley low-fat Mature Cheese** ☑

■ 1 × **Solo Slim® Low-Fat Vegetable Curry** served with a small salad and 25g grated **Rosemary Conley low-fat Mature Cheese,** followed by 1 whole papaya or large apple ☑

■ 1 × **Solo Slim® Low-Fat Moroccan Spiced Chickpea Tagine,** followed by 1 large slice of melon or 1 large apple or pear ☑

■ 1 × **Solo Slim® Low-Fat Mushroom Soup** plus 1 × **Solo Slim® Low-Fat Vegetable Curry,** followed by 1 kiwi fruit ☑

■ 1 × **Solo Slim® Low-Fat Minestrone Soup** served with 1 small wholegrain bread roll (max. 100 kcal), followed by 200g chopped melon ☑

■ 1 × **Solo Slim® Low-Fat Minestrone Soup** plus 1 × **Solo Slim® Low-Fat Vegetable Curry** ☑

■ 1 × **Solo Slim® Low-Fat Mushroom Soup** followed by 1 × **Rosemary Conley Low Gi Nutrition Bar** and 2 pieces fresh fruit ☑

■ 1 × **Solo Slim® Low-Fat Mushroom Soup** served with 1 medium slice wholegrain bread, toasted and spread with Marmite, plus 1 boiled egg, followed by 1 kiwi fruit ☑

■ 1 × **Solo Slim® Low-Fat Tomato Soup** served with 1 slice wholegrain bread, followed by 1 kiwi fruit or satsuma ☑

■ 2 slices wholegrain bread spread with very-low-fat mayonnaise made into a sandwich with salad vegetables and 30g grated **Rosemary Conley low-fat Mature Cheese** ☑

■ Toast 1 slice wholegrain bread on one side, then cover the other side with 50g grated **Rosemary Conley low-fat Mature Cheese** and place under the grill until the cheese melts. Serve with Worcestershire sauce and a small salad ☑

■ 1 × **Rosemary Conley Low Gi Nutrition Bar** plus 2 pieces fresh fruit and 1 low-fat yogurt (max. 100 kcal and 5% fat) ☑

■ 2-egg omelette made into omelette with milk from allowance, filled with 50g grated **Rosemary Conley low-fat Mature Cheese** and served with a small salad ☑

DINNERS

Approx. 400 kcal each; choose one per day

Meat and poultry dinners

■ 1 × **Solo Slim® Low-Fat Lamb Hotpot** served with unlimited vegetables (excluding potatoes), followed by 1 satsuma

■ 1 × **Solo Slim® Low-Fat Lamb Hotpot** served with 100g broccoli or cabbage or carrots plus Amazing Meringue Sundae (see recipe, p.000)

■ 1 × **Solo Slim® Low-Fat Lamb Hotpot** served with 100g new potatoes (with skins) and 100g green vegetables of your choice

■ 1 × **Solo Slim® Low-Fat Mushroom Soup** followed by 1 × **Solo Slim® Low-Fat Lamb Hotpot** served with 100g vegetables of your choice (excluding potatoes)

■ 1 × **Solo Slim® Low-Fat Beef Meatballs and Potatoes** served with 100g carrots and 100g broccoli or cabbage plus 1 × **Rosemary Conley Solo Slim® Hot Chocolate Drink** made in a cup with water or with milk from allowance

■ 1 × **Solo Slim® Low-Fat Beef Meatballs and Potatoes** served with 100g vegetables of your choice, followed by Amazing Meringue Sundae (see recipe, p.000)

■ 1 × **Solo Slim® Low-Fat Minestrone Soup** plus 1 × **Solo Slim® Low-Fat Beef Meatballs and Potatoes**

■ 1 × **Solo Slim® Low-Fat Beef Meatballs and Potatoes** served with unlimited vegetables (excluding potatoes), followed by 1 kiwi fruit

■ 1 × **Solo Slim® Low-Fat Beef Meatballs and Potatoes** served with 100g green vegetables, followed by 1 × **Rosemary Conley Low Gi Nutrition Bar**

■ 1 × **Solo Slim® Low-Fat Mushroom Soup** plus 1 × **Solo Slim® Low-Fat Chilli and Rice,** followed by 1 kiwi fruit or satsuma

■ 1 × **Solo Slim® Low-Fat Beef Casserole** served with 100g new potatoes (with skins) and unlimited vegetables (excluding potatoes)

■ 1 × **Solo Slim® Low-Fat Beef Casserole** served with unlimited vegetables (excluding potatoes), followed by Amazing Meringue Sundae (see recipe, p.000)

■ 1 × **Solo Slim® Low-Fat Tomato Soup** plus 1 × **Solo Slim® Low-Fat Beef Casserole** served with 100g broccoli

■ 1 × **Solo Slim® Low-Fat Three Bean and Chorizo Soup** plus 1 × **Solo Slim® Low-Fat Beef Casserole** served with 100g boiled green vegetables

■ 1 × **Solo Slim® Low-Fat Beef Casserole** served with unlimited vegetables (excluding potatoes), followed by 1 × **Rosemary Conley Low Gi Nutrition Bar**

■ 1 × **Solo Slim® Low-Fat Thai Chicken Curry**, followed by 1 low-fat yogurt (max. 100 kcal and 5 % fat)

■ 1 × **Solo Slim® Low-Fat Thai Chicken Curry**, followed by 1 × **Rosemary Conley Low Gi Nutrition Bar**

■ 1 × **Solo Slim® Low-Fat Thai Chicken Curry** followed by Amazing Meringue Sundae (see recipe, p.000)

■ 1 × **Solo Slim® Low-Fat Chilli and Rice** served with a side salad tossed in fat-free dressing, followed by Amazing Meringue Sundae (see recipe, p.000)

■ 1 × **Solo Slim® Low-Fat Chilli and Rice**, followed by Amazing Meringue Sundae (see recipe, page 00), plus 1 × **Rosemary Conley Solo Slim® Hot Chocolate Drink** made in a cup with water or with milk from allowance

■ 1 × **Solo Slim® Low-Fat Thai Chicken Curry** served with a large salad, followed by 1 piece fresh fruit

■ 1 × **Solo Slim® Low-Fat Thai Chicken Curry** served with 25g (dry weight) basmati rice, boiled

■ 1 × **Solo Slim® Low-Fat Chicken Hotpot** served with 100g broccoli and 100g cabbage or carrots, followed by 1 low-fat yogurt (max. 100 kcal and 5% fat)

■ 1 × **Solo Slim® Low-Fat Chicken Hotpot** served with 100g green vegetables, followed by 1 × **Rosemary Conley Low Gi Nutrition Bar**

■ 1 × **Solo Slim® Low-Fat Mushroom Soup** plus 1 × **Solo Slim® Low-Fat Chicken Hotpot** served with 100g green vegetables

■ 1 × **Solo Slim® Low-Fat Chicken Hotpot** served with 100g boiled new potatoes (with skins) plus 30g other vegetables of your choice

■ 1 × **Solo Slim® Low-Fat Pasta Bolognese** served with a large salad, followed by 1 × Hartley's Low Calorie Jelly, any flavour

■ 1 × **Solo Slim® Low-Fat Carrot and Coriander Soup** followed by 1 × **Solo Slim® Low-Fat Pasta Bolognese**

■ 1 × **Solo Slim® Low-Fat Pasta Bolognese**, followed by 1 Cadbury's Light Chocolate Mousse

Vegetarian dinners

■ 1 × **Solo Slim® Low-Fat Spicy Vegetable and Lentil Dahl** served with 1 mini pitta bread, followed by 1 × **Rosemary Conley Solo Slim® Hot Chocolate Drink** made in a cup with water or with milk from allowance ☑

■ 1 × **Solo Slim® Low-Fat Mushroom Soup** plus 1 × **Solo Slim® Spicy Vegetable and Lentil Dahl** and 1 × **Rosemary Conley Solo Slim® Hot Chocolate Drink** made in a cup with water or with milk from allowance ☑

■ 1 × **Solo Slim® Low-Fat Spicy Vegetable and Lentil Dahl** served with a small salad, followed by Amazing Meringue Sundae (see recipe, p.272) ☑

■ 1 × **Solo Slim® Low-Fat Spicy Vegetable and Lentil Dahl** served with a small salad, followed by 1 × **Rosemary Conley Low Gi Nutrition Bar** ☑

■ 1 × **Solo Slim® Low-Fat Spicy Vegetable and Lentil Dahl** served with a small salad, followed by 1 low-fat yogurt (max. 120 kcal and 5% fat) ☑

■ 1 × **Solo Slim® Low-Fat Spicy Vegetable and Lentil Dahl** served with unlimited vegetables, followed by 1 small banana ☑

■ 1 × **Solo Slim® Low-Fat Moroccan Spiced Chickpea Tagine** served with 100g vegetables of your choice, followed by 1 × **Rosemary Conley Low Gi Nutrition Bar** ☑

■ 1 × **Solo Slim® Low-Fat Moroccan Spiced Chickpea Tagine** served with unlimited vegetables of your choice (excluding potatoes), followed by 1 low-fat yogurt (max. 75 kcal and 5% fat) ☑

■ 1 × **Solo Slim® Low-Fat Moroccan Spiced Chickpea Tagine** served with a large salad, followed by 1 low-fat yogurt (max. 100 kcal and 5% fat) ☑

■ 1 × **Solo Slim® Low-Fat Moroccan Spiced Chickpea Tagine** served with 25g (dry weight) basmati rice, boiled, followed by 1 piece fresh fruit ☑

■ 1 × **Solo Slim® Low-Fat Tomato and Vegetable Pasta** sprinkled with 25g grated **Rosemary Conley low-fat Mature Cheese**, followed by 1 low-fat yogurt (max. 120 kcal and 5% fat) ☑

■ 1 × **Solo Slim® Low-Fat Tomato and Vegetable Pasta** plus 1 meringue basket filled with 1 dsp (10ml) Total 0% fat Greek Yoghurt and topped with 4 sliced strawberries or 40g raspberries ☑

- 1 × **Solo Slim® Low-Fat Tomato and Vegetable Pasta**
served with small salad tossed in fat free dressing plus
100g fresh fruit salad topped with 1 tsp Total 0% fat Greek
Yoghurt ☑
- 1 × **Solo Slim® Low-Fat Tomato and Vegetable Pasta**
served with small salad, followed by 1 × **Rosemary Conley
Low Gi Nutrition Bar** ☑
- 1 × **Solo Slim® Low-Fat Vegetable Curry** served with a
large mixed salad, followed by Amazing Meringue Sundae (see
recipe, p.000) ☑
- 1 × **Solo Slim® Low-Fat Vegetable Curry** served with 200g
vegetables of your choice (excluding potatoes), followed by 1
low-fat yogurt (max. 150 kcal and 5% fat) ☑
- 1 × **Solo Slim® Low-Fat Vegetable Curry** served with 1
blue Portion Pot® (55g dry weight) basmati rice, boiled,
followed by 1 mango, chopped ☑
- 1 × **Solo Slim® Low-Fat Three Bean Casserole** served with
1 blue Portion Pot® (55g dry weight) basmati rice, boiled ☑
- 1 × **Solo Slim® Low-Fat Three Bean Casserole** served with
70g broccoli and 70g carrots, followed by 1 low-fat dessert
(max. 135 kcal and 5% fat) or 1 × **Rosemary Conley Low Gi
Nutrition Bar** ☑
- 1 × **Solo Slim® Low-Fat Three Bean Casserole** served with
150g asparagus, followed by 1 low-fat yogurt (max. 160 kcal
and 5% fat) ☑

POWER SNACKS

Approx. 50 kcal each; choose two per day

Fruit
- 1 whole papaya, peeled and deseeded ☑
- 100g cherries ☑

- 75g fresh mango ✓
- 12 seedless grapes ✓
- 1 medium pear ✓
- 100g fresh pineapple ✓
- 1 × 200g slice melon (weighed without skin) ✓
- 150g strawberries ✓
- 1 small apple ✓
- 2 kiwi fruit ✓
- 2 dried apricots ✓
- 20g sultanas ✓
- 1 kid's fun-size mini banana ✓
- 1 kiwi fruit plus 5 seedless grapes ✓
- 2 satsumas ✓
- 2 plums ✓
- ½ grapefruit sprinkled with 1 tsp sugar ✓
- 150g fresh fruit salad ✓
- 1 red Portion Pot® (115g) raspberries plus 50g strawberries ✓
- 1 yellow Portion Pot® (70g) blueberries plus 1 tsp low-fat natural yogurt ✓
- 1 yellow Portion Pot® (125ml) fresh orange or apple juice ✓
- 1 red Portion Pot® (115g) raspberries topped with 2 tsps low-fat yogurt (max. 5% fat) ✓
- 1 × 90g pack Tesco Fresh Apple and Grape Snack Pack ✓
- 100g any stewed fruit sweetened with low-cal sweetener ✓

Sweet
- 1 fat-free yogurt, any flavour (max. 50 kcal) ✓
- 1 Hartley's Low Calorie Jelly topped with 1 tbsp Total 2% Greek Yoghurt and 3 berries of your choice
- 1 blue Portion Pot® (14g) Special K (eat dry or with milk from allowance) ✓
- 1 Caxton Pink 'n' Whites wafer ✓

Savoury

- 1 rice cake spread with 20g Philadelphia Extra Light soft cheese and sliced cucumber ☑
- 5 mini low-fat bread sticks plus 1 tsp (25g) Total 0% fat Greek Yoghurt mixed with chopped chives ☑
- 1 Asda Good For You Chicken Noodle Cup Soup
- 10 sweet silverskin pickled onions plus 10 cherry tomatoes ☑
- 20g low-fat cheese (max. 5% fat) plus 5 cherry tomatoes ☑
- 1 Rakusen's cracker topped with 1 × 20g triangle Laughing Cow Extra Light soft cheese, plus 5 cherry tomatoes
- 1 Ryvita spread thinly with Philadelphia Extra Light soft cheese ☑
- 1 Ryvita, spread with Marmite and topped with 2 tsps low-fat cottage cheese ☑
- 1 blue Portion Pot® (75g) tomato salsa plus 1 carrot, 1 celery stick and 1 × 5cm piece cucumber sliced into crudités ☑
- 2 carrots, cut into sticks, served with 1 tbsp low-fat yogurt mixed with fresh chopped chives and finely chopped red onion ☑
- 10 cherry tomatoes, plus chunks of carrots, cucumber and green or red pepper ☑
- 1 small bowl of mixed salad tossed in fat-free dressing ☑

DESSERTS

All the following desserts are 5% or less fat

Ice cream and iced desserts

- Strawberry and Rhubarb Mousse (see recipe, p.268) **125 kcal**
- 1 × 100ml serving Asda Triple Chocolate Dairy Ice Cream **101 kcal**
- 1 × 60g serving Tesco Healthy Living Banoffee Frozen Dessert **92 kcal**

- 1 × 100ml serving Wall's Soft Scoop Raspberry Ripple flavour ice cream **82 kcal** ☑
- 1 × 70g pot Marks & Spencer Count On Us Raspberry Mousse **80 kcal**
- 1 × 70g pot Marks & Spencer Count On Us Chocolate Mousse **80 kcal**
- 1 The Skinny Cow Triple Chocolate Stick **78 kcal** ☑
- 1 × 100ml serving Carte D'Or Lemon Sorbet **78 kcal**
- Tropical Sorbet (see recipe, p.267) **74 kcal** ☑
- 1 × 100ml serving Carte D'Or Light Vanilla ice cream **70 kcal**
- 1 × 100ml serving Wall's Soft Scoop Light Vanilla flavour ice cream **62 kcal**

Fruit, meringues and jelly
- Coffee and Apricot Roulade (see recipe, p.269) **108 kcal**
- 150g fresh fruit salad plus 1 tsp low-fat yogurt **100 kcal**
- Eton Mess: Break up 1 Marks & Spencer meringue basket and mix with 1 tbsp 0% fat Greek yogurt and 1 large chopped strawberry **99 kcal** ☑
- 1 Marks & Spencer meringue nest filled with 1 tbsp 0% fat Greek yogurt and topped with 1 tbsp fresh raspberries or blueberries **90 kcal** ☑
- 1 Marks & Spencer meringue basket filled with 1 tsp 0% fat Greek yogurt and topped with 1 slice pineapple, chopped **85 kcal** ☑
- 1 × 120g pot Del Monte Fruitini Fruit Pieces in juice **71 kcal** ☑
- 1 Hartley's Low Sugar Jelly plus 1 piece any fresh fruit **60 kcal**

Yogurts and fromage frais
- 1 × 200g pot Müllerlight Apricot fat free yogurt **98 kcal**
- 1 × 200g pot Müllerlight Wild Blueberry fat free yogurt **94 kcal**

■ 1 × 55g pot Asda Great Fruity Stuff fromage frais, any flavour **94 kcal** ✓

■ 1 × 125g pot Yeo Valley Organic Low Fat Raspberry Yogurt **94 kcal** ✓

■ 1 × 150g Asda Good For You Rhubarb Yogurt **91 kcal** ✓

■ 1 pot Tesco Healthy Living Lemon Cheesecake yogurt **90 kcal** ✓

■ 1 × 165g pot Müllerlight Vanilla Yogurt sprinkled with Dark Chocolate **86 kcal**

■ 1 × 125g pot Sainsbury's Be Good To Yourself Blueberry & Cranberry Fruit Yogurt **86 kcal**

■ 1 × 120g pot Danone Shape Fat Free Feel Fuller For Longer yogurt, any flavour **75 kcal** ✓

Puddings and cakes

■ Crunchy Apple and Blackberry Pie (see recipe, p.273) **139 kcal** ✓

■ Plum Tatin (see recipe, p.271) **107 kcal**

■ 1 × 100ml serving Morrisons Absolutely Gorgeous Toffee Pecan Temptation **102 kcal**

■ Banana Muffins (see recipe, p.270) **99 kcal**

■ 1 Sainsbury's Lemon Cake Slice **97 kcal** ✓

■ 1 Asda Good For You Lemon Slice **97 kcal** ✓

■ 1 Asda Good for You Cherry Bakewell Slice **96 kcal**

■ 1 Asda Good For You Chocolate Slice **95 kcal** ✓

■ 1 Mr Kipling Delightful Apple Slice **91 kcal** ✓

■ 1 Asda Good for You Carrot and Orange Cake Slice **77 kcal**

■ 1 × 100g serving Tesco Healthy Eating Summer Fruits Pudding **72 kcal**

■ 1 × ⅛ slice Soreen Lincolnshire Plum Fruit Loaf **65 kcal** ✓

TREATS

After the initial 14-day Fast Track diet, you are allowed a daily high-fat treat or alcoholic drink and a low-fat dessert (max. 100 kcal each) if your calorie allowance permits.

HIGH-FAT TREATS FOR 100 KCAL OR LESS
All the following treats are more than 5% fat.

Crisps
- 10 Pringles Lights Sour Cream & Onion flavour **99 kcal** ☑
- 1 × 21g bag Boots Shapers Salt & Vinegar Chipsticks **99 kcal** ☑
- 1 × 25g bag Walkers Baked Salt & Vinegar crisps **98 kcal** ☑
- 1 × 25g bag Jacob's Original Twiglets **96 kcal** ☑
- 1 × 18g bag Walkers Baked Wotsits Really Cheesy **95 kcal** ☑
- 1 × 19g bag Cheese & Onion Flavour Pom-Bear Teddy-shaped Potato Snacks **95 kcal** ☑
- 1 × 25g bag Walkers Squares Cheese & Onion Flavour Potato Snack **95 kcal** ☑
- 1 × 21g bag Golden Wonder Golden Lights Sour Cream & Onion crisps **94 kcal** ☑
- 1 × 21g bag Sainsbury's Be Good To Yourself 35% Less Fat Salt & Black Pepper Light & Crunchy Snacks **94 kcal** ☑
- 1 × 23g bag Walkers French Fries Ready Salted **94 kcal** ☑
- 1 × 25g bag Walkers Squares Ready Salted **94 kcal** ☑
- 1 × 24g bag Kettle Crispy Bakes Mild Cheese with Sweet Onion **91 kcal** ☑
- 1 × 18g bag Skips Prawn Cocktail snacks **89 kcal**
- 1 × 18g bag Walkers Quavers Cheese Flavour **87 kcal** ☑

Cereal bars and cakes
- 1 Cadbury Highlights Toffee Flavour Cake Bar **95 kcal** ☑
- 1 Mr Kipling Delightful Chocolate Cake Slice **95 kcal** ☑

- 1 Harvest Chewee White Choc Chip Cereal Bar **94 kcal** ☑
- 1 Kellogg's Special K Bar **90 kcal** ☑
- 1 Kellogg's Coco Pops Cereal & Milk Bar **85 kcal** ☑

Biscuits
- 2 Weight Watchers Raspberry & White Chocolate Cookies **98 kcal** ☑
- 2 Weight Watchers Double Choc Chip Cookies **98 kcal** ☑
- 3 Bahlsen Deloba biscuits **98 kcal** ☑
- 2 Sainsbury's Taste The Difference Belgian Chocolate Biscuit Thins **96 kcal**
- 3 Fox's Party Rings **93 kcal** ☑
- 1 Marks & Spencer All Butter Fruity Flapjack Cookie **95 kcal** ☑
- 2 McVitie's Jaffa Cakes **92 kcal** ☑
- 1 McVitie's Dark Chocolate HobNob **92 kcal** ☑
- 3 Rombouts Café Biscuits **92 kcal**
- 3 Cadbury Milk Chocolate Fingers **90 kcal** ☑
- 3 Lotus Original Caramelised Biscuits **90 kcal** ☑
- 1 Marks & Spencer Dutch Shortcake **90 kcal**
- 1 McVitie's Moments Chocolate Viennese Melt **90 kcal**
- 1 Tesco All Butter Traditional Scottish Shortbread Finger **90 kcal** ☑
- 4 Asda Rich Tea Fingers **88 kcal** ☑
- 1 Tesco Free From Golden Crunch biscuit **85 kcal** ☑
- 1 McVitie's Belgian Chocolate Chunk Boaster **86 kcal**
- 1 Jammie Dodgers Original **83 kcal** ☑
- 1 McVitie's Milk Chocolate Mint Digestives **81 kcal**
- 1 Green & Black's Organic Chocolate Flapjack biscuit **80 kcal** ☑
- 4 Cadbury Snaps (any flavour) **80 kcal** ☑
- 1 McVitie's Light Milk Chocolate Digestive **78 kcal** ☑
- 1 Fox's Golden Crunch Creams **75 kcal** ☑

Sweets and chocolate
- 4 Bassetts Murray Mints **100 kcal** ☑
- 1 Boots Shapers Crispy Caramel Bar **99 kcal**
- 1 × 20g fun-size bag M & Ms **98 kcal**
- 1 fun-size Twix **98 kcal**
- 1 Tesco Value Choc Ice **95 kcal**
- 2 segments Terry's Chocolate Orange **90 kcal** ☑
- 6 Cadbury Mini Eggs **90 kcal** ☑
- 1 fun-size Mars Bar **88 kcal**
- 1 mini bag Nestlé Milkybar Buttons **87 kcal**
- 1 Thorntons Mini Caramel Shortcake **86 kcal** ☑
- 4 Werther's Original **84 kcal** ☑
- 2 Galaxy Mini Eggs **80 kcal** ☑
- 1 Ferrero Rocher **75 kcal** ☑
- 1 Thorntons Continental Chocolate **70 kcal** ☑

LOW-FAT TREATS FOR 100 KCAL OR LESS
All the following treats are less than 5% fat.

Sweet treats
- 2 Caxton Pink 'n' Whites **100 kcal** ☑
- 5 Bassetts Jelly Babies **100 kcal**
- 25 Jelly Belly Jelly Beans **100 kcal**
- 10 Maynards Wine Gums Light **100 kcal**
- 24 Skittles **97 kcal** ☑
- 1 × 28g treat bag Rowntree's Jelly Tots **96 kcal** ☑
- 4 Bassetts Liquorice Allsorts **91 kcal**
- 5 Starburst Twisted Chews **90 kcal** ☑
- 5 Haribo Tangfastics **85 kcal**

Savoury treats
- 1 × 25g bag Sainsbury's Be Good To Yourself Sea Salt & Cracked Black Pepper Pretzel Sticks **95 kcal**

- 1 × 25g pack Marks & Spencer Mini Salted Pretzels **94 kcal**
- 1 × 30g bag Ryvita Minis Salt & Vinegar **93 kcal**
- 1 × 25g bag Morrisons Eat Smart Sea Salt Pretzels **87 kcal**
- 1 × 25g bag Marks & Spencer Count On Us Sour Cream & Chive Baked Potato Crisps **85 kcal**
- 1 × 25g bag Marks & Spencer Count On Us Lightly Salted Baked Potato Crisps **85 kcal**
- 1 × 20g pack Asda Good For You Crispy Cracker Selection Hickory Smoked Barbecue Flavour **76 kcal**
- 1 × 20g pack Asda Good For You Crispy Cracker Selection Sun-Dried Tomato and Herb Flavour **76 kcal**
- 1 × 20g pack Asda Good For You Crispy Cracker Selection Thai Style Sweet Chilli Flavour **76 kcal**
- 1 × 25g bag Marks & Spencer Count On Us Smokey Bacon Potato Hoops **60 kcal**
- 1 × 18g pack Ryvita Limbos Cheese & Onion **63 kcal** ☑
- 1 × 18g pack Ryvita Limbos Smokey Bacon **63 kcal** ☑
- 1 × 18g pack Ryvita Limbos Salt & Vinegar **62 kcal** ☑

ALCOHOLIC DRINKS

From Week 3 you are allowed one alcoholic drink per day up to 100 calories. Use Slimline or low-calorie mixers with spirits to keep the calories down. Here is a quick guide to calories.

Beer and cider (per 300ml/½ pint)
Bitter 91 kcal
Cider (dry) 100 kcal
Guinness 90 kcal
Lager 82 kcal

Brandy and liqueurs (per 25ml measure)
Brandy 50 kcal
Cointreau 78 kcal
Grand Marnier 78 kcal
Southern Comfort 81 kcal
Tia Maria 75 kcal

Spirits (per 25ml measure)
Bacardi 56 kcal
Gin 50 kcal
Rum 50 kcal
Vodka 50 kcal
Whisky 50 kcal

Vermouth (per 50ml measure)
Martini Extra Dry 48 kcal
Martini Rosso 70 kcal

Wine (per yellow Portion Pot®/125ml)
Champagne 95 kcal
Red wine 85 kcal
Rosé wine (medium) 89 kcal
White wine (dry) 83 kcal
White wine (medium) 93 kcal

Fortified wine (per 50ml measure)
Dry sherry 58 kcal
Sweet sherry 68 kcal
Port 79 kcal

13 The Solo Slim 28-day fitness challenge

As well as working out with me on rosemaryconley.tv for the muscle-toning sessions that are recommended on six days a week in order for you to maximise your weight loss on the Amazing Inch Loss Plan, you will need to undertake some form of aerobic exercise on six days a week. There are many forms of exercise that you may choose to undertake, but for simplicity I have set out for you a daily aerobic challenge as part of the 28-day plan. This could be anything from walking up and down stairs consecutively or going for a 30-minute brisk walk. The recommendations for each day are progressive, so please make the effort to do them. By the end of the 28-day plan you will find yourself able to do significantly more exercise than you could a month earlier.

After an exercise session, it's good to stretch out the main muscles that you have been using, to prevent soreness later. It's worth learning and remembering the leg stretches on pp.343–347 and do them after you've undertaken any activity that challenges your leg muscles. The stretches for the muscles worked in the toning workouts are included each day as we work out together on rosemaryconley.tv. Just log on to www.rosemaryconley.tv/ailpDay1, ailpDay2, etc. for the toning workouts as you continue day by day on the Solo Slim diet. These workouts are progressive, so always do them one day at a time in the correct order. See chapter 10 for details of how to progress once you have completed 28 days.

Do each stretch slowly and take care to get into the correct position, otherwise the stretch won't be effective in releasing the build-up of lactic acid that can cause aching muscles a day or two later. Hold each stretch in the extreme position for the count of 8–10 seconds and then release. You only need do each stretch once.

If you have a pedometer, wear it every day to check how active you are. Aim to achieve 10,000 steps a day, or at least 2000 more steps than your usual number, as this will help you to lose your excess weight and also to maintain it once you have achieved a healthy weight.

DAY 1

Go for a brisk 20-minute walk.

DAY 2

Walk up and down stairs 3 times consecutively. Do this 4 times in total throughout the day.

DAY 3

Work out at an aerobics class or to a fitness DVD for 30 minutes or go for a brisk 30-minute walk.

DAY 4

Go for a cycle ride for 20 minutes or cycle on a stationary exercise bike for 10 minutes, plus either walk briskly for 30 minutes at some point in the day or go for a 20-minute swim.

DAY 5

Select one of the following or create a combination of activities that you can do one after the other for a minimum of 30 minutes in total:

- Swimming
- Brisk walking
- Cycling
- Aerobics (class or DVD)
- Heavy housework (vacuuming, cleaning windows, bed making, etc.)
- Cardio equipment in the gym (e.g. stepper, cross trainer, bike, treadmill).

DAY 6

Go for a brisk walk for 20–30 minutes at some point during the day.

DAY 7

Take a brisk 30-minute walk or work out to a fitness DVD for 30 minutes. Also, walk up and down stairs 4 times consecutively, twice during the day. Really go for it today!

DAY 8

Rest day.

DAY 9

Go for a brisk walk or a swim or a bike ride for 30 minutes.

DAY 10

Do 40 minutes of aerobic work, choosing one of the following activities:
- Working out to a fitness DVD or at an aerobics class
- Swimming
- Cycling
- Brisk walking
- Use the cardio equipment at the gym (e.g. stepper, treadmill, cross-trainer, exercise bike).

DAY 11

Walk up and down stairs 4 times consecutively and repeat 4 times during the day.

DAY 12

Go for a brisk 30-minute walk and aim to clock up at least 10,000 steps on your pedometer. Alternatively, walk up and down stairs 5 times consecutively and repeat later in the day.

DAY 13

Work out for 30–40 minutes at an aerobics class or to one of my aerobic fitness DVDs (my *Real Results Workout* DVD is a great fat burner). Alternatively, go for a 40-minute brisk walk. Don't forget to stretch afterwards.

DAY 14

Take a 30–40-minute brisk walk or work out to a fitness DVD for 30–40 minutes.

DAY 15

Rest day.

DAY 16

Power walk for 30 minutes, swinging your bent arms as you walk. Increase the pace now that you are slimmer and fitter!

DAY 17

If you have a skipping rope, try skipping for as long as you can. March on the spot to give you a chance to get your breath back, then skip some more!

DAY 18

Walk up and down stairs 5 times consecutively, then repeat later in the day. In addition, go for a 15-minute brisk walk or work out at a class or to a fitness DVD.

DAY 19

Go for a 20-minute brisk walk, then skip for 5 minutes (if you have a skipping rope). Cool down by marching on the spot for 2 minutes before doing your stretches.

DAY 20

Work out energetically to a fitness DVD for 30 minutes or go for a 30-minute brisk walk.

DAY 21

Try and work out for an hour today. Salsacise, aerobics, a class, swimming energetically, working out to a DVD, using cardio equipment at the gym – they all use extra calories and they all burn fat. Drink plenty of water before, during and after your workout.

DAY 22

Rest day.

DAY 23

Work out at an aerobics class or do a fitness DVD for 40 minutes, or go for a 40-minute brisk walk, or jog for 20 minutes, or walk up and down stairs 5 times consecutively and repeat 3 times throughout the day.

DAY 24

Go for a power walk and intersperse some jogging steps even if you manage only 20 or so. Try to keep going for 30 minutes.

DAY 25

Go swimming, cycling, jogging, or anything that causes you to become mildly breathless. Try and work out for 30 minutes and remember to do your stretches at the end (see p.343–7).

DAY 26

Choose any physical activity you like that is going to make you slightly breathless but one that you can sustain for 45 minutes.

DAY 27

Do a 40-minute aerobic workout at a class or do a fitness DVD or go for a 60-minute brisk walk. Don't forget to stretch at the end.

DAY 28

Walk up and down stairs 5 times consecutively twice during the day, plus take a 40-minute power walk or jog or work out to a fitness DVD. Really go for it!

Post-aerobic stretches

1 Calf stretch

Place one foot in front, with both feet pointing forward (hold on to a wall or sturdy surface for support if you wish). Bend front knee in line with ankle and keep back leg straight with heel pressing down. Lean further forward to feel a stretch in calf of the back leg and hold for 10 seconds. Do the lower calf stretch on p.344 before changing legs.

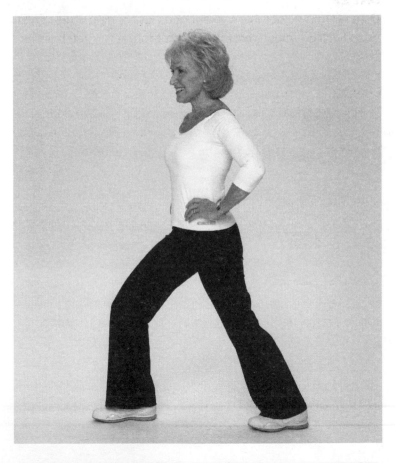

2 Lower calf stretch

Bring your back foot half a step in and bend both knees with feet still pointing forward. Keep both heels on floor and your body upright as you look straight ahead and hold for 10 seconds. Change legs and repeat both calf stretches.

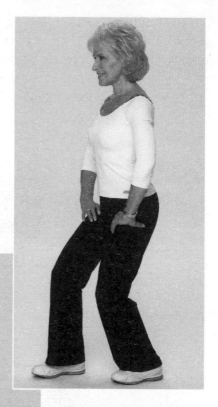

3 Back thigh stretch

Straighten your front leg and keep your back leg bent. With spine straight, lean forward slightly to feel a stretch in back thigh of straight leg. Hold for 10 seconds, then change legs and repeat.

4 Front of hip stretch

Bend front leg and lift heel of back foot. With your weight equally distributed between both legs, trunk upright and tummy in, press pelvis forward to feel a stretch at top of hip. Hold for 10 seconds, then change legs and repeat.

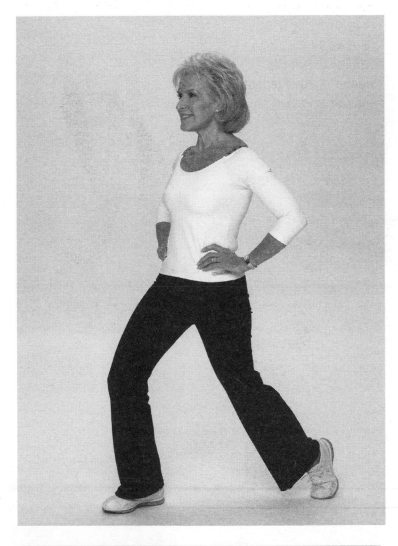

5 Front thigh stretch

Stand upright and take hold of one ankle with hand (place other hand on wall or back of chair for support if necessary). Bring knees in line with each other and keep the supporting leg slightly bent. Gently push hip of raised leg forward to stretch front of thigh. Hold stretch for 10 seconds, then change legs and repeat.

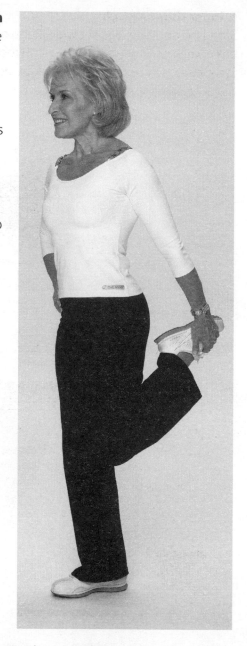

6 Inner thigh stretch

Stand tall and take legs out wide. Bend one knee in line with ankle, keeping other leg straight with foot pointing forward, to feel a stretch in inner thigh of straight leg. Hold for 10 seconds, then change legs and repeat.

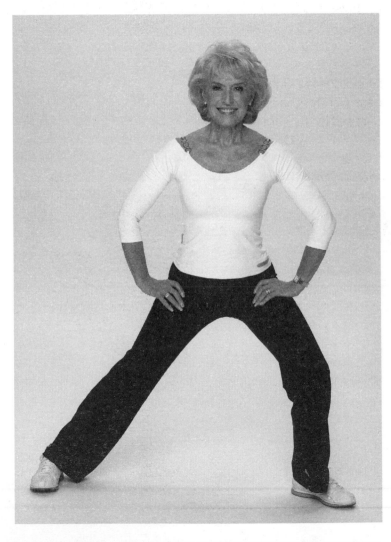

14 Are you doing your five-a-week?

We all know we should be eating our five-a-day fruit and veg but how many of us are getting enough exercise?

Wouldn't it be great if there was one thing that we could do to lower our cholesterol and blood pressure, halve our risk of heart disease and Type 2 diabetes and help protect us against some cancers and conditions like arthritis, depression and asthma? Well, there is. It's exercise!

We often complain that we don't have time for physical activity and yet in Britain we watch an average of 27 hours a week of television – that's almost four hours a day! But when we hear the Department of Health's recommendations that we should take 30 minutes of exercise five times a week, it just seems too much to fit in – and I can understand that.

We're all too busy living our lives – working, doing domestic chores, gardening, shopping, feeding, relaxing, playing, entertaining and sleeping. I believe that most of us have a 'will' to exercise and we understand that it's really good for us. The problem is *doing* it, because we just can't seem to find that 30 minutes five times a week to improve our health and wellbeing.

However, I believe there's a quicker and easier way to achieve the same benefits. It doesn't have to be 30 minutes five times a week if the activity that you do is more energetic – such as jogging, cycling, aerobics, skipping. It's all about intensity. The 'harder' you exercise, the less you need to do to achieve the same physical benefits. So, you could jog for 14 minutes or skip with a rope for eight minutes and it would be just as beneficial to your health as a half-hour walk. Or you might prefer cycling for 12 minutes but it needs to be at a rate of 13 mph if you're only doing 12 minutes. If you go to a Rosemary Conley class your 45 minutes of aerobic exercise would more than equal an hour of brisk walking, so that would count as two of your five-a-week.

Alternatively, you could break up the activities into shorter stints. A 15-minute walk would count as half of one of your five-a-week and you can fit that in as and when you have time. Just add all your activities together at the end of the week.

And don't think that exercise, to count as one of your five-a-week, has to be formal exercise such as in the gym or at a class. Washing the car, mowing the lawn, doing the vacuuming, or shovelling snow all count as exercise. They all increase our heart rate for a while and that's crucial, and they all involve using our muscles. This is what physical activity is all about and from where the benefits are derived.

Once we realise that our 'five-a-week' activity sessions don't *have* to be done in units of 30 minutes' duration, the challenge of actually doing five physical activities in a week becomes much more achievable. The next bit of good news is that our exercise doesn't *have* to be done on five separate days either to be beneficial to our health. If you wanted to do three of your five-a-week on one day and two on another, that's fine!

With this in mind, the goal of achieving our five-a-week becomes eminently do-able. So long as we challenge our heart and lungs through physical activity on a regular basis, the health benefits are life-changing and life-saving! And I'm not being over-dramatic. Taking exercise on a regular basis can have a monumentally beneficial effect on our health.

So how could *your* five-a-week look?

Rowing on a machine or jogging for 14 minutes on Monday + **aerobics** (class or DVD) on Tuesday (= 45 minutes so that counts as **two**) + general **housework** for 30 minutes on Thursday + eight minutes **skipping** on Sunday and we're there. We've done our **five-a-week**! That is totally achievable even in the busiest of lives.

How I get *my* five-a-week

Whenever I do radio or press interviews, I'm nearly always asked how much I work out each day. As I'm slim and reasonably fit people assume I must be sweating it out in the gym for two hours a day. But nothing could be further from the truth!

Until recently, my weekly fitness routine went something like this: I teach two classes on a Monday evening, which, together, usually involves up to one hour of aerobics, so that was a good two of my five-a-week. Then on Saturday or Sunday, Waise (my dog) and I went for a good walk (around three miles), which notched another two of my five-a-week. Finally, I aimed to fit in one more physical activity each week – I've just taken up ice skating and when I go it is for an hour. Now, I'm only a beginner so I'm not going to build up a sweat, but over those 60 minutes I would say it equates to two of my five-a-week. Sometimes I work out to one of my DVDs or go on the rowing machine for 15 minutes – though that's rare.

And that was it, until two bouncing black Labrador pups (BB and Sky) arrived on the scene. I now walk them around our garden every morning, to encourage outdoor toilet training. Not only does it allow them to burn off some of their boundless energy, it gets *me* moving more. I'm out with them for around 30 minutes and even though the walk is more of an amble rather than a brisk one, I have enjoyed amazing health benefits and have never felt so fit and well in my life. It's fantastic! Getting up at 6.15 every morning (except Sundays when Mike does the early shift) and walking around holding my cup of tea has now become part of my life and I'm loving it. It is such a wonderful time of the day to be outside and I really look forward to it. Waise (pronounced Visor) thinks it's great, too, and has become the perfect 'auntie' to BB and Sky.

Getting *your* five-a-week

It's all about moving more and elevating your heart rate for a while on a regular basis so that your heart becomes stronger and fitter. Alongside your heart, lungs, muscles, joints, bones and organs, and even your mind, the health benefits from the increased blood supply circulating around your body are huge. It is what your body needs – desperately!

The list below gives you a breakdown of some of the activities you might easily accommodate within your lifestyle. The key to your success is doing a form of exercise you really enjoy. If it's fun, you won't want to miss it. Do any of these activities or sports for the duration stated, even if you do them in two shorter sessions, and you can count it as one of your five-a-week.

Plan ahead what you want to do and put it in your diary or calendar. Involve the family. Tick the activities off when you've done them. You'll be amazed how quickly you will feel healthier – and how your weight loss speeds up!

FIVE-A-WEEK ACTIVITIES
Bowling 30 mins
Gardening (moderate) 30 mins
Hand washing the car 30 mins

Mopping floor 30 mins
Vacuuming 30 mins
Walking (3 mph pace) 30 mins
Window cleaning 30 mins
Ballroom dancing 25 mins
Golf (walking, pulling clubs) 25 mins
Table tennis 25 mins
Tai chi 25 mins
Aerobics/Salsa dancing (low impact) 20 mins
Aqua aerobics 20 mins
Gardening (heavy) 20 mins
Tennis (doubles) 20 mins
Waxing car 20 mins
Swimming (at 25m per minute pace) 18 mins
Cycling (at 10 mph) 17 mins
Badminton 15 mins
Hiking 15 mins
Ice skating 15 mins
Stair climbing 15 mins
Step aerobics (6-inch step) 15 mins
Tennis (singles) 15 mins
Football 14 mins
Hockey 14 mins
Jogging (at 5 mph) 14 mins
Aerobics (high impact) 14 mins
Rowing machine 14 mins
Squash 12 mins
Cross country skiing 10 mins
Cycling (at 13 mph) 10 mins
Snow shovelling 10 mins
Swimming (at 50m per minute pace) 10 mins
Skipping with rope 8 mins

Five steps to get you started

■ Assess your starting fitness level and decide which activities you could manage.

■ Plan your programme for the week and write it down.

■ Do you have the equipment to be able to achieve them? For instance, do you have a skipping rope if skipping is on your list? Do you have proper trainers to wear if you plan to jog or run? Is your bike in good order with the tyres pumped up? Does your swimsuit fit?

■ Get started and place a tick alongside your planner with details of the date, time taken, and how you felt afterwards.

■ Monitor your progress by timing yourself or measuring your distance or by wearing a pedometer.

Five ways to fit exercise into your life

■ Make the most of your time at home, e.g. get up earlier, make housework count by doing it in a proper session rather than in bits and bobs which don't raise your heart rate for long enough.

■ Involve the whole family with your five-a-week campaign. Buddy-up with each other and enjoy quality time together, chatting and having a laugh while exercising. Race each other, set challenges and score points – the one to reach the chosen target first wins a prize. Make it fun!

■ Make your physical activity a social event. Walk or jog with a friend. Work out to a DVD with a few friends in your living room or in your lunch break at work.

■ Stair climbing is a fantastic way to get fitter fast. Use the stairs as often as you can as it is great for your legs as well as your heart and lungs. Going up and down stairs five or ten times consecutively is a really effective workout and will transform your fitness level in no time.

- Walk rather than drive when you can. Even a 15-minute walk counts as half of one of your five-a-day, so build these walks into your everyday life, too.

Five ways to keep it up
- Write down what activities you plan to do at the beginning of each week.
- Select activities you enjoy.
- Mix with active people who may join in or at least encourage you.
- Be flexible and don't beat yourself up if occasionally you have to miss a session.
- If you manage to complete your five-a-week every week for a month/three months/six months, reward yourself and if the family have joined in, reward the family too!

Healthy living
The five-a-day message to encourage eating more fruit and vegetables has now become part of our healthy eating lifestyle and we all know that it is good for us even though the physical wellbeing benefits may not always be obvious to us. However, introduce the five physical activities a week into your lifestyle, too, and not only will you be amazed how quickly you feel energised, but you will sleep better, your blood pressure will reduce, your cholesterol levels will go down and your general health will benefit massively. Combine this with a healthy diet and lose a few pounds and suddenly you will feel like a new person. So, go on, just do it!

15 Eating out on a diet

Eating out is one of life's treats and there's no need to turn down a special invitation just because you are trying to lose weight. The key is to choose carefully from the menu and, with this in mind, you might find the information on the following pages helpful in steering you towards lower-calorie and lower-fat options that still taste good.

If you know you've overindulged on any particular occasion, just compensate the next day by increasing your exercise level and burning some extra calories. Walk or run more than usual or do an extra workout at a class or work out to a fitness DVD.

Please don't get hung up about having the occasional overindulgent evening, as sometimes it can help you to get back on track with the diet with extra determination and dedication. However, don't weigh yourself on the day after you've had your meal out because you will be thoroughly disheartened if you find you've gained weight. Any weight gain on such an occasion, though, is likely to be fluid rather than actual fat. Eating spicy, high-fat foods, as well as giving us loads of unnecessary calories, can cause us to retain fluid and give a false and depressing reading on the scales. If you get straight back on the diet and increase your activity levels, you'll be amazed how you 'get away' with having that delicious meal out.

During your meal, drink alcohol in moderation only, as not only does it have lots of calories, it will quickly weaken your willpower. Alcohol is also dehydrating, which is bad for your health and general wellbeing, and it will leave you exceedingly thirsty throughout the night. Try to pace your drinking by alternating a glass of wine with a glass of sparkling water. This is what I try and do and it really works, as often we just want to be holding a glass and taking a sip rather than knocking back the alcohol.

Don't be frightened of asking the waiter to serve your vegetables or any accompaniments without fat and for any dressings to be served separately on the side. Many restaurants are happy to do this and, with careful control, you can save yourself hundreds of calories and grams of fat without eating less food.

Here's a quick guide to restaurant and fast-food choices with recommendations on choosing healthier, low-fat options so you can enjoy your food without ruining your diet. All figures given for calories and fat are approximate.

Ten Tips for Dining Out

1 Plan ahead for the day of your meal out. Make an effort to reduce your calorie intake for the rest of your meals that day and save up your treat and alcohol allowance.

2 Try to avoid buffets – it's too tempting to overeat in the effort to get your money's worth. If it can't be avoided, make healthier choices and resist going back for more.

3 Before your meal, sip low-calorie drinks such as water or slimline mixers to help fill you up.

4 Avoid the bread roll, as it will have around 130 calories – and that figure will double if you add butter! Select a fruit-based starter, such as melon or sorbet, or a light soup. These options will give you few calories but help fill you up.

5 Choose main dishes that are grilled, steamed or baked, and avoid anything fried, deep-fried or sautéed. If you are not sure how something is cooked, or its ingredients, ask.

6 Don't be afraid to request a special order – ask for salads without dressings and vegetables without sauces.

7 If you want an indulgent pudding, then save up some of your treat calories. Otherwise, choose sorbets, yogurt or fresh fruit salad.

8 Enjoy a glass or two of wine but drink plenty of water in between sips.

9 Alcohol calories soon add up – so save up your alcohol allowance for a few days beforehand and keep track of what you are drinking.

10 Don't worry if you have overindulged a little – it's not the end of the world. Just cut back on the calories the next day and be more active.

Pub grub

Comfort food is key when it comes to pub grub. Pies, stodgy stews with dumplings, burgers, fish and chips, bangers and mash, Sunday roast and ploughman's lunch have all become pub regulars. Bear in mind that a pub gourmet beef burger can rack up over 1,800 calories and a Ploughman's lunch 1,146 calories! Many of the dinners and puddings may also be high in salt and bad for your cholesterol and blood pressure.

GOOD CHOICES

Starters
- Melon: 60 kcal per 200g serving 1% fat
- Tomato soup: 140 kcal per 200g serving 4% fat

Mains
- Venison in red wine sauce: 287 kcal per 300g serving 9% fat
- Lancashire hotpot: 400 kcal per 300g serving 7% fat

Desserts
- Fruit salad: 106 kcal per 200g serving 1% fat
- Summer fruit pudding: 251 kcal per 200g serving 2% fat

Other good choices:
- Smoked salmon
- Grapefruit cocktail
- Pork and apple casserole
- Shepherd's pie
- Fish pie
- Beef casserole
- Sorbet

DISHES TO AVOID

Starters
- Paté and toast: 577 kcal per 200g serving 20% fat
- Breaded mushrooms with garlic dip: 352 kcal per 150g serving 12% fat
- Chicken wings with BBQ sauce: 465 kcal per 200g serving 11% fat

Mains
- Scampi and chips: 954 kcal per 300g serving 57% fat
- Mixed grill with chips: 1,372 kcal per 300g serving 66% fat
- Steak and ale pie with chips: 1,362 kcal per 300g serving 46% fat

Desserts

- Chocolate fudge cake: 744 kcal per 200g serving 47% fat
- Sticky toffee pudding with custard: 688 kcal per 200g serving 24% fat

Other dishes to avoid:

- Prawn cocktail
- Avocado starter
- Ploughman's lunch
- Beef Wellington
- Sausage and mash
- Toad in the hole
- Gammon steak and chips
- Beef stew with dumplings
- Beefburger
- Sponge pudding and custard
- Ice-cream sundae
- Treacle tart and custard
- Fruit crumble and custard
- Apple pie and custard
- Spotted dick and custard

Pub snack watch

It can be easy to notch up a load of calories and fat simply by indulging in some snacks from behind the bar. Check out the calorific snacks below:

- 40g pork scratchings: 285 kcal 54% fat
- 100g McCoys crisps: 504 kcal 29.2% fat
- 100g salted peanuts: 622 kcal 53% fat

Pub grub tips

■ Avoid fried foods.

■ Avoid dishes with creamy or rich sauces and ask for them to be served separately.

■ Steer clear of any dishes with pastry, e.g. pies.

■ Go for dishes that are grilled, poached or chargrilled.

■ Trim any visible fat from meat and chicken.

■ Opt for a jacket potato, new potatoes or salad instead of chips.

■ Ask for vegetables to be served without butter, and salad without dressing.

■ Avoid cheese.

Italian

Whether it's pizza or pasta, Italian food is notoriously high in carbohydrates, and choosing lower-calorie, lower-fat options isn't always easy. An average portion of lasagne contains about 650 kcal and 44g fat. Some Italian chains and restaurants now offer lighter options, but these can still be laden with calories and fat. For instance, a typical salad with dressing can contain more calories than a medium pizza.

GOOD CHOICES

Starters

■ Minestrone soup: 152 kcal 3.5g fat per 200g serving

■ Rocket and pecorino salad (rocket leaves with shavings of pecorino cheese): 163 kcal 4.5g fat per 300g serving

Mains

■ Chargrilled medium pizza (thin base): 709 kcal 28.2g fat per medium pizza

■ Arrabiata pasta: 441 kcal 13.1g fat per 450g serving

Desserts
■ Fresh fruit salad: 89 kcal 0.6g fat per 200g serving
■ Granita di limone (lemon water ice): 119 kcal 0.3g fat per 200g serving

Other good choices:
■ Mixed side salad (no dressing)
■ Napoletana pasta
■ Pasta bolognese
■ Grilled fish
■ Chicken Caesar salad (with dressing served separately)
■ Fresh fruit salad
■ Lemon sorbet

DISHES TO AVOID

Starters
■ Antipasto: 547 kcal 34.7g fat per 200g serving
■ Mozzarella tomato salad: 542 kcal 48.8g fat per 300g serving

Mains
■ Pepperoni medium pizza (deep base): 1,764 kcal 95.4g fat per pizza
■ Pollo pasta with pesto: 983 kcal 27.7g fat per 450g serving

Desserts
■ Tiramisu: 448 kcal 20.6g fat per 150g
■ Profiteroles: 571 kcal 46.9g fat per 150g

Other dishes to avoid:
■ Bruschetta
■ Cannelloni
■ Calamari (fried)

- Lasagne
- Carbonara pasta
- Alfredo pasta
- Pepperoni calzone
- Parmesan cheese (it's 33% fat)
- Noci (walnuts)
- Zabaglione
- Banoffee pie
- Cheesecake

Italian food tips

- Avoid pasta with creamy sauces such as alfredo and carbonara.
- Choose pasta or baked dishes with tomato-based sauces such as arrabiata, Napoletana, marinara, and pomodori rather than fried or creamy ones.
- Give garlic bread a miss.
- Avoid *permigiana* dishes – they are floured, fried and baked with cheese.
- Go easy on dishes with pesto – they contain olive oil.
- Choose thin-crust pizzas like 'Tuscani' rather than deep pan and ask for less cheese on top.
- Go for healthy pizza toppings such as chicken, tuna and vegetables – but resist the olive oil.
- Avoid high-fat pizza toppings such as pepperoni, salami, anchovies and olives.
- Share a pizza and have a side salad (no dressing).

Mexican

With calorific sour cream, guacamole, refried beans and cheesey dishes on the menu, Mexican menus can be a dieting minefield. Most restaurant chains have adopted the American-style nacho cheese dishes and many side dishes are high in fat (a side portion of refried beans could contain around 350 calories and 30% fat!). Huge portions seem to be hard to avoid and one meal could push you over your full day's calorie allowance. However, the meat is normally flame-grilled or barbecued rather than fried, saving on fat and calories, and many of the fattening sauces and dips are often served separately, so it's easier to avoid these extra calories.

GOOD CHOICES

Starters
■ Ceviche (citrus marinated fish): 128 kcal per 200g serving 2% fat
■ Quinoa salad: 215 kcal per 140g serving 4% fat

Mains
■ Vegetable fajitas (grilled vegetables, served with salsa without the sour cream, guacamole and cheese): 428 kcal per 350g serving (2 fajitas) 6% fat
■ Chicken burrito (no cheese): 572 kcal per 350g serving 4% fat
■ Chicken fajitas (grilled chicken, served with salsa without the sour cream, guacamole and cheese): 467 kcal per 350g serving 9% fat

Desserts
■ Fruit mess (guava, or other fruit, natural yogurt, and crushed meringue): 180 kcal per 200g serving 3% fat
■ Sorbet margarita: 114 kcal per 150g serving 0% fat

Other good choices:
■ Brown rice
■ Soft tacos with beans and salsa

- Mexican stew
- Shrimp ceviche

DISHES TO AVOID

Starters
- Chicken quesadilla (tortilla, cheese and chicken): 428 kcal per 200g serving 36% fat
- Nachos (with cheese, guacamole, salsa and sour cream): 523 kcal per 200g serving 50% fat

Mains
- Beef tacos (crispy tortilla with salsa, sour cream, guacamole, rice, beef and cheese): 703 kcal per 350g serving (2 tacos) 22% fat
- Vegetable chimichanga (fried tortilla with salsa, guacamole, sour cream, rice, refried black beans and roast vegetables): 752 kcal per 350g serving 24% fat
- Beef enchiladas (tortillas with cheese, beef, sautéed onions and peppers baked in the oven and topped with melted cheese): 842 kcal per 350g serving 54% fat

Desserts
- Sopaipillas (fried dough with cinnamon and honey): 530 kcal per 200g serving 13% fat
- Capirotada (Mexican bread pudding): 571 kcal per 200g serving 31% fat

Other dishes to avoid:
- Enchiladas (stuffed tortilla covered in cheese)
- *Tamales* (dough filled with pork or chicken, wrapped in maize leaves and steamed)

- Flautas (small rolled-up tortilla filled with beef or chicken and fried)
- *Chile relleno* (fried chilli pepper stuffed with melting cheese and meat)
- *Tostadas* (flat or bowl-shaped tortilla that is toasted or deep-fried)
- Mexican burgers
- Chilli con carne
- Fries

Mexican food tips

- Opt for barbecued or grilled meats.
- Look for chicken or vegetable fillings.
- Salsa is virtually fat-free and has about 18 calories per 50g serving. So choose salsa to accompany dishes instead of sour cream, guacamole and refried beans which are all high in fat and calories.
- When in doubt choose a soft tortilla-based meal over the crunchy variety which are fried – this will save you hundreds of calories.
- Avoid ordering extra chips, potato wedges or onion rings as most meals are large enough and already have accompaniments.
- Mexican restaurant portions are often massive – try to share meals or don't be afraid to leave leftovers once you're full.

Indian

Indian food has become a firm favourite, with its flavoursome, hot and spicy curries, different types of bread and tasty chutneys. The problem is that most of the dishes are prepared with ghee (clarified butter) or coconut oil and milk, making them high in fat. Britain's most popular curry dish – chicken tikka masala (which didn't even originate from India) is definitely a curry to avoid for dieters. Watch out, too, for deep-fried side dishes and starters and even some types of rice and breads.

However, a lot of Indian cuisine includes healthy grains and vegetables so look out for those on the menu. Indian dishes are also perfect for sharing, so just keep tabs on how much you've eaten and you can still enjoy a healthier curry that's full of flavour.

GOOD CHOICES

Starters
- Poppadom with raita (cucumber dip): 65 kcal per 12g serving 18% fat
- Yellow dahl (yellow lentils): 172 kcal per 200g serving 3% fat

Mains
- Vegetable balti: 290 kcal per 500g serving 2% fat
- Tandoori chicken : 426 kcal per 500g serving 1.5% fat
- Chicken tikka: 459 kcal per 500g serving 2% fat

Desserts
- *Kesari*: 217 kcal per 150g serving 5% fat
- Mango sorbet: 151 kcal per 150g serving 0% fat

Other good choices:
- Lentil soup
- Paneer tikka
- Lime pickle
- Onion salad
- Chapati or roti bread
- Jalfrezi
- Rogan josh

- Tandoori fish
- Curried vegetables
- Boiled or steamed basmati rice
- Dahl
- Cucumber salad
- Fresh fruit

DISHES TO AVOID

Starters
- Beef samosas: 335 kcal per 50g serving (2 medium) 13.2% fat
- Onion bhaji: 838 kcal per 150g serving 48% fat

Mains
- Chicken biryani: 985 kcal per 500g serving 9% fat
- Chicken korma: 855 kcal per 500g serving 11% fat
- Chicken tikka masala: 1,146 kcal per 500g serving 22% fat

Desserts
- Gulab jamun (dumplings in sweet syrup): 632 kcal per 150g serving 20% fat
- Kulfi (Indian ice cream): 426 kcal per 150g serving 13% fat

Other dishes to avoid:
- Naan or paratha
- Saag paneer
- Samosas
- Korma
- Masala
- Pakora
- Pasanda
- Dupiaza
- Fried rice
- Panir (made with Indian cheese)

Indian food tips

- Portions can be generous, so share a main course with a friend.
- Ask for poppadoms to be grilled rather than fried.
- Choose tandoori or tikka dishes (without additional sauces) as these tend to be grilled or barbecued rather than fried.
- Opt for chicken- and prawn-based dishes – they are lower in fat than lamb.
- Choose tomato-based dishes such as jalfrezi and rogan josh rather than cream-based ones such as korma, masala or pasanda.

Watch those sides

Indian side dishes are often loaded with calories and fat. Here's some of the best and worst on the menu.

- Pilau rice   582 kcal per portion
- Aloo saag   354 kcal per portion
- Bombay potatoes   350 kcal per portion
- Naan bread   300 kcal per bread
- Boiled rice   245 kcal per portion
- Chapati   197 kcal per bread

Chinese

Traditional Chinese cuisine is typically fresh and healthy with a balance of flavours such as hot and cold, pickled and fresh, spicy and mild. But the western take on Chinese food has resulted in high-calorie, fat-laden noodle and rice dishes and deep-fried accompaniments. Moreover, many dishes are fried in oil so meals that seem relatively healthy are often packed with fat and calories.

But there are still many healthy and tasty options such as dim sum, steamed rice, fish, chicken and vegetable dishes. Be sure to choose sauces and side dishes carefully and check the way that the meat or veg is cooked. Portions are generous so order one starter, one main and a rice dish to share with a friend.

GOOD CHOICES

Starters
- Chicken and sweetcorn soup: 110 kcal per 215g serving 5% fat
- Prawn wonton: 80 kcal each 3% fat

Mains
- Beef in hoisin sauce: 340 kcal per 250g serving 11% fat
- Chicken with beansprouts: 275 kcal per 250g serving 9% fat

Desserts
- Mandarin sorbet with lychees: 163 kcal per 150g serving 1% fat
- Mango pudding: 140 kcal per 150g serving 0% fat

Other good choices:
- Dim sum (if stewed or steamed)
- Tofu (steamed or baked)
- Meat or vegetables with hoisin sauce
- Beef with black bean sauce
- Stir-fried bamboo shoots, water chestnuts or spring greens

DISHES TO AVOID

Starters
- Crispy duck: 400 kcal per 2 pancake serving 22% fat
- Sesame prawn toasts: 328 kcal per 150g serving 26% fat

Mains
- Pork balls with sweet and sour sauce: 1,136 kcal per 10 balls serving 48% fat
- Cashew chicken: 536 kcal per 250g serving 44% fat

Desserts
- Banana fritters: 556 kcal per 150g serving 36% fat
- Eight treasures rice pudding: 330 kcal per 150g serving 13% fat

Other dishes to avoid:
- Spring rolls
- Crispy seaweed
- Dim sum (fried)
- Ribs
- Crispy Peking duck (no skin)
- Crispy lamb
- Sweet and sour dishes
- Chicken chow mein
- Deep-fried vegetable dishes

Chinese food tips
- Choose sauces such as black bean or hoisin as these are lighter and generally lower in fat and calories than other sauces.
- Opt for steamed or stir-fried dishes – they'll fill you up but with less fat.
- Eat with chopsticks – the meal will last longer and be much more fun.
- Avoid deep-fried dishes such as spring rolls, seaweed and prawn toast.
- Stay away from sweet and sour dishes. The meat is often deep-fried and the sauces are high in sugar and therefore calories.

- Avoid dishes with cashew nuts – they are over 50% fat. Beware of prawn crackers – they contain 10 calories each and are 35% fat.

Watch those sides

Chinese side dishes are often heavy on calories and fat, so take a look at these to see the best and worst on the menu:

- Special fried rice   630 kcal per portion
- Egg fried rice   625 kcal per portion
- Singapore fried noodles   529 kcal per portion
- Boiled rice   320 kcal per portion
- Boiled noodles   315 kcal per portion
- Bamboo shoots   80 kcal per portion

Tapas

Tapas are tasty small dishes that originate from Spain and are becoming more popular as an eating out option. In Spain, tapas were commonly nibbled as appetisers or a snack before a session of drinking or a meal, but now they take on many forms and can be practically anything based around olives, chorizo, seafood, potato and vegetables.

Tapas can be deceiving for the dieter because while the portions are small, dishes are usually cooked in large amounts of olive oil, making the fat content sky high.

However, a tapas menu has a large range of food on offer, so there's a variety of healthy options.

GOOD CHOICES

- *Ensalada verde mixta* (green salad with feta cheese, cucumber, radishes, carrots and lettuce): 73 kcal 9.6g fat per 180g serving

- *Pimiento relleno* (peppers stuffed with rice, onion, tomato, herbs and cod): 128 kcal 6.2g fat per 200g serving
- Paella: 215 kcal 5.4g fat per 200g serving
- Pisto (similar to ratatouille with a mixture of squash, onions, garlic and tomatoes): 79 kcal 3.9g fat per 200g serving
- Marinated calamari: 97 kcal 2.4g fat per 77g serving

Desserts
- Fresas frescas (fresh strawberries): 56 kcal 0.2g fat per 200g serving

Other good choices:
- *Escalibada* (grilled or barbecued vegetables)
- Gazpacho (cold soup)
- Salmon Español (Spanish salmon)
- Chicken sofrito (stir-fried chicken)
- *Olla podrida* (chickpea and pork stew)
- *Cocida Gallego* (meat stew with vegetables)
- *Judias verdes cos jamón* (green beans with ham)
- *Bacalao a la Vizcaina* (salt cod with tomatoes, onions and green peppers)
- *Melon y jamón Serrano* (fresh melon slices topped with Serrano ham)

DISHES TO AVOID

- Salted almonds: 327 kcal 25g fat per 80g serving
- Battered shrimps: 241 kcal 5.4g fat per 200g serving
- Deep-fried calamari: 234 kcal 12g fat per 77g serving
- *Chorizo al vino* (Spanish sausage fried in red wine): 740 kcal 61.6g fat per 200g serving
- *Pescado blanco frito* (deep-fried white fish): 486 kcal 37.8g fat per 200g serving

Desserts

■ Churros (hot fritters): 395 kcal 13.8g fat per 200g serving

Other dishes to avoid:

■ Chorizo (spicy Spanish paprika sausage)
■ Garlic shrimps
■ *Calamares a la Romana* (deep-fried squid rings)
■ *Escabeche* (spicy cold dish of fish or poultry – fried then marinated)
■ *Pollo Marbella* (chicken, cooked with paprika, chorizo, sweet peppers and cream sauce)
■ Sweet pastries
■ *Crema Catalana* (vanilla custard with caramelised sugar)

Tapas tips

■ Avoid anything that says 'fritta' (this means fried) or 'a la plancha' (pan fried).
■ Don't over order – limit yourself to a certain number of dishes and remember to share them!
■ Go for baked dishes with tomato-based sauces rather than fried or creamy ones.
■ Spanish Serrano ham is a great alternative to chorizo.
■ Go easy on Spanish omelette as it may be cooked in olive oil
■ If you're a newcomer to tapas, many restaurants offer set menus for two, but make sure you know which dishes to avoid and don't be afraid to ask for alternatives.

16 Maintaining your new weight

Once you have arrived at your ultimate goal weight, you'll want to maintain your new, slim figure and you may be worrying about what to do next.

Eating

To avoid weight gain, you need to continue with the low-fat, low-Gi, principles of eating. If you have found that eating more protein is helpful, then carry on with this. If you go back to eating high-fat snacks, cooking with fat and using fatty or oily dressings on your food, you will only pile back on the fat that you've worked so very hard to lose. Just as you can wean yourself away from the taste of high-fat foods, it is easy to retrain yourself back into your old, bad habits again and, if you do, you will regret it. This doesn't mean that you can't ever have a cream cake, a packet of crisps or a Big Mac. Of course you can. But only occasionally and it needs to be seen as a treat, and an exception rather than the rule.

Depending on your age and weight you can increase your calories by a couple of hundred calories a day and stick to that for the next three or four weeks. Then, if you can keep your weight stable at that level, you can increase the calories a little more and see if you are able to keep your weight constant. If you find the weight starts to creep back on, cut down again. Or if you have overindulged, for instance after a holiday or Christmas break, you can return to the 14-Day Fast Track diet, or use my Solo Slim® foods for a week to shift your excess weight. You may find yourself tempted to stay on such a low level of calories, but this is unwise as you will find that after a while your willpower will break and you'll eat for Britain! Trust me, just use it as a booster occasionally.

If you are aged 60 or over, you will not be able to eat more than about 1500 calories a day without putting on weight unless you do a lot of exercise. Hopefully, you will fall into a routine that allows you to eat enough and stay slim without feeling that you are dieting. Try to relax and gradually you will build your self-confidence in controlling your eating.

Another great way to help you maintain your new weight is to eat relatively 'normally' throughout the week, but select two days each week when you either return to the Fast Track Fortnight diet or eat Solo Slim® foods (see page 304). This will give you two days a week when you cut your calories right back to 1200 a day, which will then allow you that little bit of freedom if you want to eat more calories over the weekend. This works really well for some people.

For the party animals among you, you may find that you want to eat anything and everything over the weekend from Friday to Sunday and then choose to eat in a much more controlled way from Monday to Friday. Again, Solo Slim® can play a major role here and you could choose one meal a day from the Solo Slim® range to keep you on track.

The success of weight maintenance is being able to eat healthily and stay active long term without feeling that you're dieting. I don't ever feel as if I'm on a diet, but I eat healthily all the time and if I find that my waistband is getting a little tight, I just cut back on quantities for a couple of weeks, and it all gets sorted out. I also increase my activity levels, by taking our dogs for more walks – and walking a bit faster – or doing an extra workout to one of my DVDs. Just being more active on a day-to-day basis can make a massive difference to your overall calorie expenditure. If I'm trying to lose a few pounds, I will do my own errands, distributing things around the office rather than asking my PA to take them for me! I recommend that you wear a pedometer to check how many steps you are doing. I know of no better gadget for motivating you and encouraging you to move more.

Exercise

Continue with your five-a-week aerobic activity at a level that makes you mildly breathless and warm so that you achieve fat-burning mode. If you like working out to fitness DVDs, my Real Results Workout is terrific with great motivating music. It is a brilliant all-round programme and offers a 30-minute aerobic fat-burning workout, two 20-minute highly effective toning sections and two 'Express' workouts that take less than five minutes each. All my fitness DVDs – and I have recorded 30 of them – give you a fabulous fat-burning whole body workout, but the main thing is that anyone can do them, as every move is demonstrated at different levels of ability to suit both the most fit and the least fit of followers.

If you want to continue with the toning exercises designed to accompany this book, just log on to www.rosemaryconley.tv /ailpDay14, etc. and repeat the exercises recommended in the last two weeks of the 28-day programme (Day 14 through to Day 28). Work at a level that challenges you so when you are able to increase the number of reps, do so, to reach a level where you can feel mild discomfort, and then do two more.

Once you have become fitter, and your muscles are stronger and well toned, it doesn't take endless exercise to keep your body fit and trim. But if you don't use it, you will lose it!

17 Your personal calorie allowance

On the following two pages you will find tables indicating the average basal metabolic rate (BMR) of males and females, according to age and weight. The number of calories listed under the relevant calories (BMR) column tells you how many your body uses each day just to fulfil your bodily functions – if you stayed in bed all day and did nothing, your body would still burn this number of calories. As soon as you get out of bed and start moving around, going about your everyday work and daily activities and doing some exercise, the number of calories spent increases dramatically. Eating enough calories to meet your basal (basic) metabolic needs should ensure your body receives sufficient nutrients to stay healthy. Then the additional calories that you are bound to spend by moving about and undertaking your everyday activities, will have to be taken from your fat stores, and you will lose weight.

Once you have completed the 28-day Amazing Inch Loss Plan, I recommend that you work out your daily calorie intake, as above, and then calculate your daily food intake so it falls within that number. By using the Amazing Inch Loss Plan diet as your basis for your daily eating, you can then add extra portion sizes, desserts, alcohol or low-fat treats, if your calorie allowance permits. I suggest you limit any high-fat treats to 100 calories per day (700 per week) during your weight-loss programme. Once you've reached your ideal weight, please see pages 274–292 for advice and help on maintaining your new weight long term.

Your personal calorie allowance (women)

Check against your current weight and age range to find the ideal daily calorie allowance that will give you a healthy rate of weight loss after you've completed the initial 28-day plan.

Women aged 18–29			Women aged 30–59			Women aged 60–74		
Body Weight		(BMR)	Body Weight		(BMR)	Body Weight		(BMR)
Stones	Kilos	Calories	Stones	Kilos	Calories	Stones	Kilos	Calories
7	45	1147	7	45	1108	7	45	1048
7.5	48	1194	7.5	48	1144	7.5	48	1073
8	51	1241	8	51	1178	8	51	1099
8.5	54	1288	8.5	54	1211	8.5	54	1125
9	57	1335	9	57	1220	9	57	1151
9.5	60.5	1382	9.5	60.5	1287	9.5	60.5	1176
10	64	1430	10	64	1373	10	64	1202
10.5	67	1477	10.5	67	1389	10.5	67	1228
11	70	1524	11	70	1414	11	70	1254
11.5	73	1571	11.5	73	1440	11.5	73	1279
12	76	1618	12	76	1466	12	76	1305
12.5	80	1665	12.5	80	1492	12.5	80	1331
13	83	1712	13	83	1518	13	83	1357
13.5	86	1760	13.5	86	1544	13.5	86	1382
14	89	1807	14	89	1570	14	89	1408
14.5	92	1854	14.5	92	1595	14.5	92	1434
15	95.5	1901	15	95.5	1621	15	95.5	1460
15.5	99	1948	15.5	99	1647	15.5	99	1485
16	102	1995	16	102	1673	16	102	1511
16.5	105	2043	16.5	105	1699	16.5	105	1537
17	108	2090	17	108	1725	17	108	1563
17.5	111	2137	17.5	111	1751	17.5	111	1588
18	115	2184	18	115	1776	18	115	1614
18.5	118	2231	18.5	118	1802	18.5	118	1640
19	121	2278	19	121	1828	19	121	1666
19.5	124	2325	19.5	124	1854	19.5	124	1691
20	127	2373	20	127	1880	20	127	1717

Your personal calorie allowance (men)

Check against your current weight and age range to find the ideal daily calorie allowance that will give you a healthy rate of weight loss after you've completed the initial 28-day plan.

Men aged 18–29			Men aged 30–59			Men aged 60–74		
Body Weight		(BMR)	Body Weight		(BMR)	Body Weight		(BMR)
Stones	Kilos	Calories	Stones	Kilos	Calories	Stones	Kilos	Calories
7	45	1363	7	45	1324	7	45	1232
7.5	48	1411	7.5	48	1347	7.5	48	1270
8	51	1459	8	51	1387	8	51	1307
8.5	54	1507	8.5	54	1425	8.5	54	1345
9	57	1555	9	57	1480	9	57	1383
9.5	60.5	1602	9.5	60.5	1527	9.5	60.5	1421
10	64	1650	10	64	1590	10	64	1459
10.5	67	1698	10.5	67	1640	10.5	67	1497
11	70	1746	11	70	1676	11	70	1535
11.5	73	1794	11.5	73	1713	11.5	73	1573
12	76	1842	12	76	1749	12	76	1611
12.5	80	1890	12.5	80	1786	12.5	80	1649
13	83	1938	13	83	1822	13	83	1687
13.5	86	1986	13.5	86	1859	13.5	86	1725
14	89	2034	14	89	1895	14	89	1763
14.5	92	2082	14.5	92	1932	14.5	92	1801
15	95.5	2129	15	95.5	1968	15	95.5	1839
15.5	99	2177	15.5	99	2005	15.5	99	1877
16	102	2225	16	102	2041	16	102	1915
16.5	105	2273	16.5	105	2078	16.5	105	1953
17	108	2321	17	108	2114	17	108	1991
17.5	111	2369	17.5	111	2151	17.5	111	2028
18	115	2417	18	115	2187	18	115	2066
18.5	118	2465	18.5	118	2224	18.5	118	2104
19	121	2513	19	121	2260	19	121	2142
19.5	124	2561	19.5	124	2297	19.5	124	2180
20	127	2609	20	127	2333	20	127	2218

Index of recipes

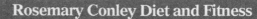

Find out more about what we do!

"Come and explore our website to see how we can inspire, motivate, advise and energise you!"

Rosemary Conley CBE

The complete weight loss solution

Log onto our website to see the great ways in which you can lose or maintain your weight!

www.rosemaryconley.com